# DELEGATION OF NURSING CARE

## Patricia Kelly-Heidenthal, RN, MSN
Professor Emerita
Purdue University Calumet
Hammond, Indiana

## Maureen T. Marthaler, RN, MSEd
Assistant Professor of Nursing
Purdue University Calumet
Hammond, Indiana

THOMSON
DELMAR LEARNING

Australia   Canada   Mexico   Singapore   Spain   United Kingdom   United States

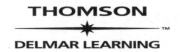

Delegation of Nursing Care
by Patricia Kelly-Heidenthal, RN, MSN, and Maureen T. Marthaler, RN, MSEd

**Vice President of Health Care Business Unit:**
William Brottmiller

**Editorial Director:**
Cathy L. Esperti

**Acquisitions Editor:**
Melissa Martin

**Marketing Director:**
Jennifer McAvey

**Channel Manager:**
Tamara Caruso

**Editorial Assistant:**
Patricia M. Osborn

**Production Editor:**
John Mickelbank

Library of Congress Cataloging-in-Publication Data

Kelly-Heidenthal, Patricia.
 Delegation of nursing care / Patricia Kelly-Heidenthal, Maureen T. Marthaler.
  p. ; cm.
  Includes bibliographical references and index.
  ISBN 1-4018-1405-0 (alk. paper)
  1. Nursing Care—Personnel management.  2. Nursing services—Administration.  3. Delegation of authority.  I. Marthaler, Maureen T. II. Title.
  [DNLM: 1. Nursing care—organization & administration—United States.  2. Delegation, Professional—legislation & jurisprudence—United States.  3. Delegation, Professional—organization & administration—United States. WY 100 K297d 2005]
 RT89.3.K45 2005
 362.17′3′068—dc 22
                                      2004049801

ISBN 1-4018-1405-0

# CONTENTS

# CONTRIBUTORS

**Rinda Alexander, PhD, RN, CS**
Professor of Nursing
Purdue University Calumet
Hammond, Indiana
Professor of Nursing
University of Florida
College of Nursing
Gainesville, Florida

**Margaret M. Anderson, EdD, RN, CNAA**
Associate Professor and Chair
Department of Nursing and Health Professions
Northern Kentucky University
Highland Heights, Kentucky

**Ida M. Androwich, PhD, RNC, FAAN**
Professor, Community, Mental Health and Administrative Nursing
Niehoff School of Nursing
Loyola University Chicago
Chicago, Illinois

**Deloris Armstrong, RN, BSN**
Senior Project Coordinator,
SETON Healthcare Network
Magnet Hospital
Austin, Texas

**Anne L. Bernat, RN, MSN, CNAA**
Consultant
Arlington, Virginia

**Sister Kathleen Cain, OSF, JD**
Attorney
Franciscan Legal Services
Baton Rouge, Louisiana

**Corinne Haviley, RN, MS**
Director, Ambulatory Care Services
Northwestern Memorial Hospital
Chicago, Illinois

**Paul Heidenthal, MS**
Consultant
Austin, Texas

**Karen Houston, RN, MS**
Director Quality and Continuum of Care
Albany Medical Center
Albany, New York

**Mary Anne Jadlos, MS, ACNP-CS, CWOCN**
Acute Care Nurse Practitioner
Wound, Skin, Ostomy Service
Northeast Health Acute Care Division
Troy, New York

**Stephen Jones, MS, RNC, PNP, ET**
Pediatric Clinical Nurse Specialist/Nurse Practitioner
The Children's Hospital at Albany Medical Center
Albany, New York
Founder, Pediatric Concepts
Averill Park, New York

**Glenda Kelman, PhD, ACNP-CS**
Chairperson, Division of Nursing
The Sage Colleges, Troy, New York
and Acute Care Nurse Practitioner
Wound, Skin, Ostomy Service
Northeast Health Acute Care Division,
Troy, New York

**vii**

**Mary Elaine Koren, RN, DNSc**
Assistant Professor
School of Nursing
Northern Illinois University
DeKalb, Illinois

**Lyn LaBarre, MS, RN, CEN**
Nurse Manager, Emergency
Department
Albany Medical Center
Albany, New York

**Linda Searle Leach, PhD, RN,
CNAA**
Assistant Professor of Nursing
California State University
Fullerton, California

**Camille B. Little, MS, RN**
Instructional Assistant Professor
Mennonite College of Nursing at
Illinois State University
Normal, Illinois

**Sharon Little-Stoetzel, RN, MS**
Assistant Professor of Nursing
Graceland University
Independence, Missouri

**Patsy L. Maloney, RNC, MSN, EdD,
CNAA**
Associate Professor and Director
Continuing Nursing Education
School of Nursing
Pacific Lutheran University
Tacoma, Washington

**Judith W. Martin, RN, JD**
Attorney
Franciscan Legal Services
Baton Rouge, Louisiana

**Mary McLaughlin, RN, MBA**
Project Specialist
Albany Medical Center
Albany, New York

**Terry W. Miller, PhD, RN**
Dean and Professor
School of Nursing, Pacific Lutheran
University
Tacoma, Washington
Professor Emeritus
San Jose State University, California

**Leslie H. Nicoll, PhD, MBA, RN**
Consultant
Editor-in-Chief
*Computers in Nursing*
Editor
*Journal of Hospice and Palliative Nursing*
Portland, Maine

**Laura J. Nosek, PhD, RN**
Adjunct Associate Professor of Nursing
Frances Payne Bolton School of
Nursing
Case Western Reserve University
Cleveland, Ohio
and
Course Facilitator, Graduate Teaching
Faculty
Excelsior College
Albany, New York

**Amy Androwich O'Malley, RN,
MSN**
Director of Nursing Resources
Children's Memorial Hospital
Chicago, Illinois

**Karin Polifko-Harris, PhD, RN,
CNAA**
Vice President for System Development
and Research
Naples Community Healthcare System
Naples, Florida

**Robyn Pozza, JD**
Attorney
Austin, Texas

**Jacklyn L. Ruthman, PhD, RN**
Assistant Professor
Bradley University
Peoria, Illinois

**Patricia M. Lentsch Schoon,
MPH, RN**
Assistant Professor
College of St. Catherine
St. Paul, Minnesota

**Kathleen Fischer Sellers, PhD, RN**
Assistant Professor
SUNY at Utica/Rome
Utica, New York

**Janice Tazbir, RN, MS, CCRN**
Assistant Professor
Purdue University Calumet
Hammond, Indiana

# REVIEWERS

Diane H. Blanchard, Ph.D., RN, CNS,
  SANE
Assistant Professor of Nursing
Alcorn State University
Natchez, Mississippi

Teresa Bryan, RN, MSN
Assistant Professor of Nursing
Alcorn State University
Natchez, Mississippi

Cindy McCoy, RN, Ph.D., MSPH,
  CEN
Associate Professor of Nursing
Northern Kentucky University
Highland Heights, Kentucky

Danielle L. White, RN, MSN
Associate Professor
Austin Peay State University
School of Nursing
Clarksville, Tennessee

Lucy White
Assistant Professor of Nursing
Ivy Tech State College
Terre Haute, Indiana

Denise York, RN, C, CNS, MS, Med
Associate Professor of Nursing
Columbus State Community College
Columbus, Ohio

# PREFACE

*Delegation of Nursing Care* is designed to help nursing students develop the knowledge, skill, and competency to delegate nursing care quickly, efficiently, and safely. The book is written by two nursing authors with special contributions from a malpractice lawyer, Robyn D. Pozza. There are many contributors and references in the book from nurse faculty, nurse administrators, nurse managers, nurse lawyers, and so on. These contributions are from authors in various areas of the United States, such as Illinois, Indiana, Louisiana, New York, Texas, and Washington, thus illustrating a broad view of nursing delegation.

*Delegation of Nursing Care* is designed to educate nursing students about the delegation process and to supply the practicing nurse with practical information about delegation. In developing this text, we have integrated information from hundreds of articles and books from nursing, business, and the social sciences.

Safe delegation is critically important to nurses and patients. In the 1960s, nurse educators emphasized clinical skills and total patient care nursing, where the nurse managed the care of a few patients. Unfortunately, skill in delegation was not emphasized and a generation of nurses was educated with very little knowledge or practical experience with delegation. The recent nursing shortage has highlighted the need to change this. This book discusses the importance of nursing delegation as one of the skills a nurse needs for quality patient care. A list of patients appear before chapter one. The patients are included in scenarios throughout the book to build knowledge and critical thinking skills.

Each chapter discusses the latest information relevant to its specific topic. Chapters contain case studies, nursing or health care quotes, interviews, stop and think exercises, and literature applications, all designed to enhance the student's learning. Within each chapter, various points of view are presented through interviews with staff nurses, nursing administrators, physicians, and others. At the end of each chapter, there is a section of exploring the web exercises, NCLEX style review questions, review activities, references, and suggested readings.

# ORGANIZATION

*Delegation of Nursing Care* consists of five chapters. These five chapters provide beginning nurses with the delegation expertise needed to succeed in today's health care environment. The chapters are arranged as follows:

Chapter One introduces the concept of delegation and applies it to nursing care of patients. Concepts of assignment, supervision, accountability, authority, responsibility, critical thinking, decision-making, as well as organizational responsibility for patient care and the chain of command are discussed.

Chapter Two discusses the National Council of State Boards of Nursing Delegation Decision-Making Grid, the Five Rights of Delegation, the role of State Boards of Nursing in Delegation, sources of power, and delegation responsibilities of health team members. The National Council of State Boards of Nursing Grid highlights the elements of decision-making that the nurse uses in delegating care. The five Rights of Delegation emphasize elements the nurse uses to maintain safety for patients when delegating care. Power is explored as an important requirement for the nurse in developing delegation ability.

Chapter Three discusses effective communication. Nurses need effective communication skills to work with patients and health care members of different cultures. The need for safe delegation emphasizes the importance of clear communication even more. This chapter also discusses the professional role of the nurse, potential barriers to communication, Myers-Briggs Personality Types, and other elements of workplace communication.

Chapter Four discusses time management and setting priorities. Nurses use time management and priority setting skills constantly when delegating care. The nurse constantly assesses, evaluates, and re-assesses and re-evaluates patient care and safety when delegating care. The nurse identifies time wasters, learns to use time well, make efficient shift reports, and make patient care assignments. Time management and priority setting assist with this process.

Chapter Five discusses legal aspects of patient care and delegation. The nurse considers legal aspects of delegating patient care and maintains patient safety with ethical behavior and by avoiding common malpractice areas. This chapter discusses malpractice cases reported from July 2001 through July 2002 and identifies a nursing checklist to decrease the risk of liability.

The textbook uses tables, figures, and photographs to engage learners and enhance their knowledge development. These tables, figures, and photographs provide visual reinforcement of concepts such as delegation, communication, time management, setting priorities, and the legal aspects of nursing.

# CHAPTER FEATURES

The chapters include several features that provide the learner with a consistent format for learning and an assortment of resources for understanding and applying the knowledge presented here.
These features include:

- A photo that begins each chapter and establishes the visual background for the reader's approach to the chapter.

- Quotes from a nursing or health care leader.

- Real world interviews that demonstrate various points of view on content.

- Stop and think exercises that encourage the reader to think critically about the content.

- Review questions, written in NCLEX style that test the student's knowledge of important content.

- Review activities that encourage the student to build on the chapter content by applying the information to their nursing activities.

- Case studies that encourage students to think critically about how to apply chapter content to the workplace and other "real world" situations. Case studies provide reinforcement of key delegation skills.

- Web exercises, which guide the student with Internet addresses for the latest information related to the textbook's content.

- References, which are the key for students to find sources of the material presented in the text.

- Suggested readings, which help the students find additional information concerning the topics covered in the text.

- Glossary terms are in **bold** type throughout each chapter. The glossary is designed to encourage understanding of new terms presented in the chapter and a complete glossary appears at the end of the text.

- Literature applications, which link current literature to practice.

- Tables and figures, which appear throughout the text and provide convenient information for the student's reference.

- A list of patient descriptions is before chapter 1 and is referenced in scenarios throughout the book to build critical thinking and decision-making skills.

# ACKNOWLEDGMENTS

Many people must work together to produce any book. A book such as this requires much effort and the coordination of many people with various areas of expertise. I would like to thank all of the contributors for their time and effort in sharing their knowledge gained through years of experience in clinical, academic, and legal settings. I thank the reviewers for their time spent critically reviewing the manuscript and providing the valuable comments that have aided this text.

I would like to acknowledge and sincerely thank the team at Delmar Publishers who have worked to make this textbook a reality. Matt Filomonov, Acquisitions Editor, is a great person who has worked tirelessly and brought knowledge, guidance, humor, and attention to help keep me motivated and on track throughout the project. Thanks to Patricia Osborn, Editorial Assistant, who also supported me every step of the way.

Thanks go to my co-author, Maureen T. Marthaler, and also to Robyn D. Pozza for being such a pleasure to work with. Thanks also to Deloris Armstrong and Dr. Patricia Padjen for their content suggestions and critical reviews and to the nurses and staff in Austin, Texas, who contributed forms, interviews, many good ideas, and much support to this project. These include Bonnie Clipper Salzberg, Deborah Duncan, Sue Thompson, Lorraine Flatt, Jerry Van den Honert, Carla Case, Shawna Sadlier, Connie Behrhorst, Joe Sanchez, Carl King, Brenda Vega, Mark Dorward, Jan Robinson, Jan Costley, Chris Curtis, Mary Lowery, Connie Faircloth, Lorraine Chandler, Karen Woodard, Ana Zeletz, Lisa Lilly, Elena Stockton, Martha Lichenhan, and Nels Arnston, St. David's Hospital, Austin, Texas; and Joyce Batchellor, Colleen Mullins, Karen Burkman, Seton Healthcare Network, Austin, Texas; and Ramona Hamilton, computer consultant, Austin, Texas, for all their help on this project.

## SPECIAL THANKS

A special thank you goes to Paul Heidenthal, for helping me with every stage of the book. Special thanks to my Aunt Pat Kelly, who encouraged me to start writing books. Special thanks also go to my parents, Ed and Jean Kelly, my sisters, Tessie Dybel and Kathy Milch, Aunt Verna and Uncle Archie Payne, Aunt Pat and Uncle Bill Kelly, to my nieces, Natalie Bevil, Melissa Arredondo, and Stacey Milch, and nephew, John Milch, and my grand nephew, Brock Bevil,

**xvii**

to my dear friends, Patricia Wojcik, Florence Lebryk and Lee McGuan, who have supported me through this book and most of my life. Special thanks to my wonderful nursing friends, Zenaida Corpuz, Dr. Mary Elaine Koren, Dr. Barbara Mudloff, Dr. Patricia Padjen, Jane McKeon, and especially to Gerri Kane, Janice Klepitch, Sylvia Komyatte, Julie Martini, Judy Rau, Anna Fizer, Carol Mihalso Lukasik, Trudy Keilman Walters, Georgia Zacny Gradek, Judy Ilijanich, Ivy Schmude, Lillian Rau, Mary Kay Moredich, and others who have supported me throughout this book and during our 40 years together as nurses. Special thanks to my faculty mentors, Dr. Imogene King, Dr. Joyce Ellis, and Nancy Weber.

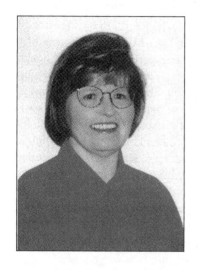

Patricia Kelly-Heidenthal earned a Diploma in Nursing from St. Margaret Hospital School of Nursing, Hammond, Indiana; a baccalaureate in nursing from DePaul University in Chicago, Illinois; and a master's degree in nursing from Loyola University in Chicago, Illinois. She has worked as a staff nurse and as a school nurse. Pat has traveled extensively, teaching conferences for the Joint Commission on Accreditation of Healthcare Organizations. She was director of quality assurance for nursing at the University of Chicago Hospitals and Clinics in Chicago, Illinois.

Pat has taught at Wesley-Passavant School of Nursing, Chicago State University, and Purdue University Calumet in Hammond, Indiana. She is Professor Emerita, Purdue University Calumet, Hammond, Indiana. Pat has taught fundamentals of nursing, adult nursing, nursing leadership and management, nursing issues, nursing trends, and legal aspects of nursing. She has taught nursing conferences in almost every state in the United States, as well as in Puerto Rico and Canada on quality improvement. Pat also teaches NCLEX reviews nationally with Health Education Systems, Inc., and is a member of Sigma Theta Tau and the American Nurses Association. She is listed in *Who's Who in American Nursing, 2000 Notable American Women,* and the *International Who's Who of Professional and Business Women.*

Pat has served on the Board of Directors of Tri City Mental Health Center, St. Anthony's Home, and Mosby's Quality Connection. She is the editor and author of *Nursing Leadership and Management,* Delmar, 2003; *Essentials of Nursing Leadership and Management,* Delmar, 2004; and she contributed a chapter entitled "Preparing the Undergraduate Student and Faculty to Use Quality Improvement in Practice" to *Improving Quality,* Second Edition, by Claire Gavin Meisenheimer, Aspen, 1997. Pat has written several articles, including "Chest X-Ray Interpretation" and many articles on quality improvement. Pat is a disaster volunteer for the American Red Cross and volunteers at a church food pantry in Austin, Texas. Throughout much of her career, she has taught nursing at the university level and has continued to work part time as a staff nurse in the Emergency Department. This has allowed her to wear several hats and see nursing from many points of view. Pat currently lives in Austin, Texas, and can be reached at patkh1@aol.com.

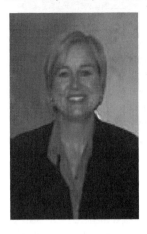

Maureen T. Marthaler earned a baccalaureate degree in nursing from Lewis University in Romeoville, Illinois, and a master's degree in nursing education from DePaul University in Chicago. She taught at Prairie State College in Chicago Heights, Illinois. Currently, Maureen is an assistant professor at Purdue University Calumet in Hammond, Indiana. Maureen has taught fundamentals of nursing, adult nursing, nursing leadership and management, nursing ethos, and critical care nursing courses. She has taught nursing conferences on various neurological conditions, such as assessment, seizures, Guillian-Barré, Parkinson's Disease, and blood gas assessment. Maureen has also taught NCLEX reviews nationally. She is the treasurer for Mu Omega Chapter of Sigma Theta Tau and is a member of the National League for Nursing.

Maureen contributed a chapter on delegation of nursing care to the Kelly-Heidenthal textbook published by Delmar, *Nursing Leadership and Management,* 2003. Maureen also wrote a continuing education program for Sigma Theta Tau International on delegation. Her most recent publication "SARS: What Have We Learned" in the nursing journal *Registered Nurse,* was co-authored with her colleagues at Purdue University Calumet. She has traveled to Romania and assisted a nursing school there with curriculum development. Throughout her career, she has continued to work part time as a staff nurse in the Intensive Care Unit at St. Margaret's Hospital in Hammond, Indiana.

Maureen has been licensed as an RN for over 23 years. She is married to David, a very supportive husband. She is the mother of two wonderful teenage boys, Luke, 15, and Jake, 13. They live in Crete, Illinois, where Maureen can be reached at maureen@calumet.purdue.edu.

# LIST OF PATIENT DESCRIPTIONS

The list below provides a list of patients and their status on any given day in a typical hospital setting. They are referenced in scenarios throughout the text to help the students to build critical thinking and decision-making skills.

| Room | Name | Age | Description |
|------|------|-----|-------------|
| 2501 | Joe Zagone | 25 | Patient admitted last night with HIV and pneumonia, has a WBC count of 3,000. |
| 2502 | Pat Cronin | 50 | Patient admitted yesterday with cancer of the liver. Jaundiced and scheduled for insertion of a Medication Port today. Severe abdominal pain complaints. |
| 2503 | Sylvia Thomas | 66 | Patient admitted with congestive heart failure and diabetes. She takes digitalis and insulin, is noncompliant with treatment and diet, almost ready for discharge. |
| 2504 | Sue Black | 60 | Patient transferred from ICU last night with a Zoloft overdose/attempted suicide. History of depression, husband died last year. |
| 2505 | Bob Clark | 22 | Patient newly admitted with acute pancreatitis. Assumes fetal position and frequently complains of abdominal pain. |
| 2506 | Patty Homan | 61 | Patient admitted with a hypertensive crisis three days ago, blood pressure decreasing daily, now 180/102. |
| 2507 | Terry Summer | 61 | Patient admitted yesterday with chronic cholecystitis and cholelithiasis, has frequent pain complaints, currently refusing surgery. |

| Room | Name | Age | Description |
|------|------|-----|-------------|
| 2508 | Empty | | Room is empty. A patient with acute exacerbation of Chronic Obstructive Pulmonary Disease is in the ER awaiting admission. |
| 2509 | Pam Glusak | 67 | Patient transferred two hours ago from ICU with a recent brain attack/CVA, is non-responsive and has right-sided paralysis. Family at bedside. |
| 2510 | Ray Olson | 89 | Patient admitted with renal failure, confused at times, will be dialyzed soon. |
| 2511 | Helen Zurich | 78 | Patient admitted with cellulitis of the right toe and a history of diabetes mellitus, needs teaching. |
| 2512 | Bobbie Anderson | 33 | Patient admitted yesterday, scheduled for partial thyroidectomy today. |

# CHAPTER 1

The authority was delegated to me to care for this patient and, by assuming this responsibility for the patient, I will then be accountable for this patient's care.
(Phyllis Franck and Marjorie Price, 1980)

# Concept of Delegation

## OBJECTIVES

*Upon completion of this chapter, the reader should be able to:*

1. Discuss concepts of delegation, assignment, supervision, accountability, authority, and responsibility.
2. Describe Benner's Model of Novice to Expert.
3. Discuss types of delegation.
4. Review obstacles to delegation.
5. Discuss organizational responsibilities for delegation.
6. Review the chain of command.
7. Identify elements of critical thinking and decision-making.

*Sue Black was admitted to the hospital with a Zoloft overdose and suicide attempt. After she was stabilized in the Intensive Care Unit (ICU), she was transferred to the Medical Surgical Unit, Room 2504. Mary, RN, was assigned to her care. A sitter, Jane, was delegated to stay with her at all times per hospital policy. As the day shift went on, the sitter asked Mary, the RN, to be relieved for lunch. Mary agreed to send an unlicensed assistive personnel (UAP) to relieve Jane for lunch.*

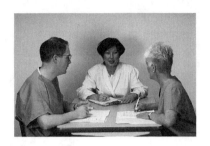

- *What are the responsibilities of Mary, Jane, and the UAP?*
- *Who is accountable for Sue Black's safety?*

(See patient description, p.xxi)

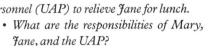

According to the American Nurses Association (ANA) Code of Ethics for Nurses with Interpretive Statement, (ANA, 2001) the nurse is responsible and accountable for individual nursing practice and determines the appropriate delegation of tasks consistent with the nurse's obligation to provide optimum patient care.

A priority responsibility for nurses is to deliver safe patient care. To ensure that this responsibility is met, nurses are accountable under the nurse practice act for patient care delivered by both themselves and other personnel under their supervision. These personnel may include other registered nurses (RN), licensed practical/vocational nurses (LPN/LVN), and UAP. UAP is an umbrella term applied to many categories of unlicensed assistive personnel such as nurse aides, nurse technicians, patient care technicians, nurse support personnel, nurse extenders, personal care attendants, unit assistants, nursing assistants, and other non-licensed personnel. UAP are trained to function in an assistive role to the licensed registered nurse in providing patient care activities as delegated by the nurse (ANA, 1992). Note that in some states, healthcare assistive personnel are licensed.

This chapter will discuss the concepts of delegation, assignment, supervision, accountability, authority, and responsibility. It will also discuss Benner's Model of Novice to Expert, concepts of critical thinking and decision making, types of delegation, obstacles to delegation, organizational responsibility for delegation, and the chain of command.

## PERSPECTIVES ON DELEGATION

Florence Nightingale is quoted as saying, "But then again to look to all these things yourself does not mean to do them yourself. . . . But can you not insure that it is done when not done by yourself? (Nightingale, 1859, p. 17). Nursing delegation was discussed by Nightingale in the 1800s and has continued to evolve since then. Delegation is needed because of the advent of cost containment, the shortage of nurses, increases in patient acuity levels, an elderly chronic population, and advances in health care technology.

Today, delegation is a must for the new nurse as well as for the experienced nurse. Benner's (2000) work reminds us that nurses need information and the opportunity for skill building in delegation, especially at the start of their career. See Table 1-1.

Delegating to personnel with different educational levels from a variety of nursing educational programs requires nurses to be vigilant and ensure that

## TABLE 1-1
### *BENNER'S MODEL: NOVICE TO EXPERT*

| Benner's Model: Novice to Expert | Application to Delegation |
| --- | --- |
| Novice nurses are recognized as being task oriented and focused on the rules. They tend to see nursing as a list of tasks to do rather than seeing the bigger picture of total patient care needed to meet patient care goals. Once novices have mastered most tasks required to perform their ascribed roles, they move on to the phase of advanced beginner. | The novice nurse is new to the direct patient care setting. The novice may have been educated in principles of delegation but has not used them in the clinical setting. Novices are task oriented, focused on perfecting their own skills, and are often still in orientation. Novices may begin to delegate tasks clearly outlined by the hospital, for instance, they may ask UAP to distribute drinking water to patients but they often cannot decide what else to delegate. The novice tries to do all the tasks without help and may be slow to recognize abnormal physical and diagnostic findings, supervise others who provide care, perform psychomotor skills, and respond to emergencies. |
| The advanced beginner is the nurse who can demonstrate marginally acceptable independent performance. This nurse still focuses on the rules but is more experienced. The advanced | This nurse is out of orientation and has worked for just a short while on the unit. The advanced beginner is able to perform most nursing tasks that are required for patient care. This nurse is becoming more |

*(continues)*

**Table 1-1**  (*continued*)

| | |
|---|---|
| beginner still needs help identifying priorities. | comfortable delegating simple tasks to UAP, such as errands, assisting in positioning of patients, bathing, and taking vital signs. He or she is often reluctant to delegate to any staff whose personality is resistant to their delegation. He or she often needs to develop their organizational and time management skills and ability to manage a group of patients. Their clinical skills, teamwork, and leadership skills still need development. |
| Competent nurses have been in their role for several years. These nurses have developed the ability to see their actions as part of the long-range goals set for their patients. They lack the speed of the proficient nurse, but they are able to manage most aspects of clinical care. | Several years in the same role allows nurses to develop the ability to see their actions as part of the long-range goals set for their patients. They are delegating less skilled tasks to UAP so that the nurse is free to perform higher level skills and make judgments. The competent nurse is more able to assess the staff's abilities, communicate expectations effectively, and gather clinical information from them. This nurse is more comfortable delegating to staff even in the presence of personality conflicts. This nurse expects that all staff members must meet the requirements of their job descriptions. |
| Proficient nurses characteristically perceive the whole situation rather than just seeing a series of tasks. They have often been on the job many years. They develop a plan of care and then guide the patient from Point A to Point B. They draw on their past experiences and know that in a typical situation, a patient must exhibit specific behaviors to | Proficient nurses perceive the whole situation rather than a series of tasks. These nurses are often charge nurses developing plans of care for the whole unit. They see delegation of tasks as an important part of guiding patients from Point A to Point B. They are able to use past experiences with patients and staff to guide the delegation process. |

*(continues)*

**Table 1-1**  (*continued*)

| | |
|---|---|
| meet specific goals. They realize that if those patient behaviors are not demonstrated within a certain time frame, then the plan of nursing care needs to be changed. | |
| Expert nurses are those nurses who intuitively know what is going on with their patients. Their expertise is so embedded in their practice that they have been heard to say, "There is something wrong with this patient. I'm not sure what is going on, but you had better come and evaluate them." Not heeding the observations derived from the intuitive sense of an expert nurse has resulted in patient deterioration and subsequent cardiac arrest. These expert nurses often seek advanced education. | These nurses intuitively know what is going on with their patients and what their patients' needs are. They can quickly assess what needs to be delegated and evaluate continuously the progress of care. |

Adapted from Benner, PE, 2000. From Novice to Expert: Excellence and Power in Clinical Nursing Practice (Commemorative Edition), Upper Saddle River, NJ: Prentice Hall.

# REAL WORLD INTERVIEW

I was in a situation where I just didn't think my patient looked good. I decided to go ahead and start two new IV sites, just in case. The patient arrested two hours later and we really needed those IV sites. I felt good about my decision.

*Cheryl* Buntz, RN

safety is maintained for the patient. When delegating to all levels of nursing staff, RNs are accountable for the outcome of patient care. When delegating to UAP who are not trained in the nursing process, the RN also retains accountability for all aspects of the nursing process, including the implementation process and patient outcomes. For example, when an RN delegates the process of ambulating a patient to UAP, the RN remains accountable for assessing the patient's ability to ambulate, assuring that the patient is ambulated according to standards, and helping the patient achieve a safe outcome, that is, not allowing the patient to fall. The RN must monitor both the competency, education, and skill of the UAP and the stability of the patient needing a delegated task. This monitoring is done initially and continues throughout the task. Thus, efficient delegation protects the patient.

## Delegation

**Delegation** is defined as "the transfer of responsibility for the performance of an activity from one individual to another while retaining accountability for the outcome. Example: the nurse, in delegating an activity to an unlicensed individual, transfers the responsibility for the performance of the activity but retains professional accountability for the overall care" (ANA, 1992). Note that delegation is different than assignment.

## Assignment

**Assignment** is the downward or lateral transfer of both the responsibility and accountability of an activity from one individual to another. The lateral or downward transfer must be made to an individual of skill, knowledge and judgment. The activity must be within the individual's scope of practice (ANA, 1992).

Tasks can properly be assigned to an individual who understands the assignment, has similar skill, knowledge, and judgment, and acts within the legal authority of the regulatory scope of practice, such as another registered nurse. An example is a charge registered nurse assigning the care of four patients to a staff registered nurse. The registered nurse making the assignment is accountable for his or her decision in making the assignment. For example, it is inappropriate for the charge nurse to assign the total care of a complex patient to a new graduate nurse until the new graduate is completely oriented and prepared for the assignment. However, once the new staff nurse accepts the assignment, he or she will assume responsibility and accountability for the care of that patient. That individual is now practicing on the basis of his or her own credentials. In the true sense of the word, then, assignments can never be made to UAP (Zimmerman, 1997).

**Assignment versus Delegation.** Note that there is a significant difference between assigning care to another RN and delegating to an LPN/LVN or UAP. The assignment or delegation must fall within the individual's legal scope of practice. Experienced RNs are expected to work with minimal supervision of their nursing practice. The RN who assigns care to another competent registered nurse, who then assumes responsibility and accountability for that patient's care, does not have the same obligation to closely supervise that person's work as when the care is delegated to an LPN/LVN or UAP. The RN can delegate responsibility to the LPN/LVN or UAP, but the RN retains accountability for the patient's care. LPN/LVNs and UAP work under the direction of the RN.

Assigning full-care responsibility and accountability to a new graduate or to a nurse working in an unfamiliar specialty may be unsafe. In these instances, the supervising nurse has a greater responsibility and accountability to evaluate the abilities and performance of the new nurse (Barter & McLaughlin, 1997). Certain actions may be delegated to an LPN/LVN in keeping with the scope of practice as designated by state regulation. If the LPN is certified in IV therapy, and the policy of the state and the employing institution permits LPNs/LVNs to provide IV treatment, the RN should not have an inordinate duty to supervise the work of the LPN once the LPNs skills in this area are demonstrated. Note that prior competency certification of the LPN may have been done through a skills day or through a competency validation. This competency validation may ensure that the LPN has been observed inserting an IV successfully three times under direct supervision of an RN in states where this practice by an LPN is allowed. The RN cannot assign responsibility and accountability for total nursing care to UAP or LPNs, but the RN can delegate certain tasks to them in keeping with the job description, knowledge base, and demonstrated competency of these individuals. The RN is then responsible for adequate supervision of the person to whom the task is given (Barter & McLaughlin, 1997).

## STOP AND THINK

Steve, RN, is working with a new RN, Josie. Josie is wondering how delegation differs from assignment. Steve tells Josie that when she assigns patient care to another RN, that RN assumes both responsibility and accountability for the care. When Josie delegates to UAP, she delegates responsibility but keeps the accountability for that patient's care. When Josie asks Jill, the UAP, to give a bath, is she delegating or assigning care? What is Jill responsible for?

## Supervision

**Supervision** is the provision of guidance or direction, evaluation, and follow-up by the licensed nurse for accomplishment of a nursing task delegated to UAP (NCSBN, 1995). Supervision is generally categorized as on site (the nurse being physically present or immediately available while the activity is being performed) or off site (the nurse has the ability to provide direction through various means of written and verbal communication).

A nurse who is supervising care will provide clear directions to his or her staff about what tasks are to be performed for specific patients. The supervisor nurse must identify when and how the task is to be done and what information must be collected as well as any patient-specific information. The nurse must identify what outcomes are expected and the time frame for reporting results. The nurse will monitor staff performance to ensure compliance with established standards of practice, policy, and procedure. The supervisor nurse will obtain feedback from staff and patients and intervene, as necessary, to ensure quality nursing care and appropriate documentation.

Hansten and Washburn (1998) identify three levels of supervision, based on the task delegated and the education, experience, competency, and working relationship of the people involved. The three levels are:

- Unsupervised—occurs when one RN works with another RN. Both are accountable for their own practice.
- Initial direction and periodic inspection—occurs when an RN supervises licensed or unlicensed staff, knows the staff's training and competency level, and has a working relationship with the staff. For example, an RN who has worked with UAP for several weeks is now comfortable giving them initial directions to ambulate two new postoperative patients. The RN follows up with the UAP once and then as needed during the shift.
- Continuous supervision—occurs when the RN determines that the delegate needs frequent to continuous support and assistance. This level is required when the working relationship is new, the task is complex, or the delegate is inexperienced or has not demonstrated competency.

## Accountability

**Accountability** is being responsible and answerable for actions or inactions of self or others in the context of delegation (NCSBN, 1995). The RN is accountable for the performance of tasks delegated to others, for tasks the nurse personally performs, and for the act of delegating activities to others. When authority has been delegated and responsibility assumed, the delegate is then accountable for the delegated task. The accountability for the performance of the task becomes shared, because the delegator also remains accountable for the completion of the delegated task. The RN is accountable for monitoring changes in the patient's status, noting and implementing treatment for the patient's responses to illness, and assisting in the prevention of complications. Nursing tasks that do not involve direct patient care can be reallocated more freely and carry fewer legal implications for RNs than delegation of direct nursing practice activities (American Association of Critical Care Nurses, 1990).

In a hospital, the UAP and LPNs/LVNs are accountable to the RN. Accountability for the act of delegating involves the appropriate choice of person and activity. For example, an RN might delegate to UAP the authority to perform a certain task. If the RN has not determined in advance that the person understands the assignment and has the skills, knowledge, and judgment to fulfill the task or the RN does not supervise the task completion, and the UAP does not perform the task adequately, the RN would be accountable for this act of improper delegation.

## AUTHORITY

**Authority** is the right to act or to command the action of others. Authority comes with the job and is required for a nurse to take action. The person to whom a task and authority has been delegated must be free to make decisions regarding the activities involved in performing those tasks. Without authority the nurse cannot function to meet the needs of patients. Authority is commonly delegated to the nurse in the nurse's job description. See Figure 1-1.

Authority is based on each individual state's nurse practice act. If a nurse is in charge of a group of patients, the nurse must have the authority or the right to act or command the action of others. Note that there are four possible levels of authority to be used by the RN when delegating a task to another nurse (Cox, 1997). See Table 1-2.

An understanding of the level of authority at the time the task is delegated and the level of authority that is identified by the state nurse practice act and the agency's job description prevents each party from making inaccurate assumptions about authority for delegated assignments.

## RESPONSIBILITY

**Responsibility** is the obligation involved when one accepts an assignment. The delegation process is not complete until the person who receives the assignment accepts it. Without this acceptance of obligation or responsibility, authority cannot be delegated. Further, if a person does not have the knowledge, skill,

## ALBANY MEDICAL CENTER HOSPITAL PATIENT CARE SERVICES
### Job Description

### JOB TITLE: REGISTERED PROFESSIONAL NURSE

| | |
|---|---|
| Exempt (Y/N): No | JOB CODE: |
| SALARY LEVEL: N25.1-4 | DOT CODE: |
| SHIFT: | DIVISION: PATIENT CARE SVC |
| LOCATION: NURSING UNITS | DEPARTMENT: |
| EMPLOYEE NAME: | SUPERVISOR: NURSE MANAGER |
| PREPARED BY: AMY BALUCH | DATE: 03/22/95 |
| APPROVED BY: | DATE: |

**SUMMARY:** The Registered Professional Nurse utilizes the nursing process to diagnose and treat human responses to actual or potential health problems. The New York State Nurse Practice Act and A.N.A. Code for Nurses with Interpretive Statements guide the practice of the Registered Professional Nurse. The primary responsibilities of the Registered Professional Nurse as leader of the Patient Care Team is coordination of patient care through the continuum, education, and advocacy.

**ESSENTIAL DUTIES AND RESPONSIBILITIES** include the following. Other duties may be assigned.

—Performs an ongoing and systematic assessment, focusing on physiologic, psychologic, and cognitive status.

—Develops a goal directed plan of care that is standards based. Involves patient and/or significant other (S.O.) and health care team members in patient care planning.

—Implements care through utilization and adherence to established standards that define the structure, process and desired patient outcomes of nursing process.

—Evaluates effectiveness of care in progressing patients toward desired outcomes. Revises plan of care based on evaluation of outcomes.

—Demonstrates competency in knowledge base, skill level and psychomotor skills.

—Demonstrates applied knowledge base in areas of structure standards, standards of care, protocols and patient care resources/references. Practices in compliance with state and federal regulations.

—Demonstrates knowledge of Patient Bill of Rights by incorporating it into their practice.

*(continues)*

**Figure 1-1** Job Description (Courtesy, Albany Medical Center, hospital patient care services, job description for registered professional nurses, Albany NY)

—Demonstrates ability to identify, plan, implement and evaluate patient/S.O. education needs.

—Participates in development and attainment of unit and service patient care goals.

—Organizes and coordinates delivery of patient care in an efficient and cost effective manner.

—Documents the nursing process in a timely, accurate and complete manner, following established guidelines.

—Utilizes standards in applying the nursing process for the delivery of patient care.

—Participates in unit and service quality management activities.

—Demonstrates self-directed learning and participation in continuing education to meet own professional development.

—Participates in team development activities for unit and service.

—Demonstrates responsibility and accountability for professional standards and for own professional practice.

—Supports research and its implications for practice.

—Adheres to unit and human resource policies.

—Establishes and maintains direct, honest, and open professional relationships with all health care team members, patients, and significant others.

—Seeks guidance and direction for successful performance of self and team, to meet patient care outcomes.

—Incorporates into practice an awareness of legal and risk management issues and their implications.

**QUALIFICATION REQUIREMENTS:** To perform this job successfully, an individual must be able to perform each essential duty satisfactorily. The requirements listed below are representative of the knowledge, skill, and/or ability required. Reasonable accommodations may be made to enable individuals with disabilities to perform the essential functions.

**EDUCATION and/or EXPERIENCE:** Graduate of an approved program in professional nursing. Must hold current New York State registration or possess a limited permit to practice in the State of New York.

**LANGUAGE SKILLS:** Ability to read and interpret documents such as safety rules and procedure manuals. Ability to document patient care

*(continues)*

**Figure 1-1** *(continued)*

on established forms. Ability to speak effectively to patients, family members, and other employees of organization.

**MATHEMATICAL SKILLS:** Ability to add, subtract, multiply, and divide in all units of measure, using whole numbers, common fractions, and decimals. Ability to compute rate, ratio, and percent.

**REASONING ABILITY:** Ability to identify problems, collect data, establish facts, and draw valid conclusions.

**PHYSICAL DEMANDS:** The physical demands described here are representative of those that must be met by an employee to successfully perform the essential functions of this job. Reasonable accommodations may be made to enable individuals with disabilities to perform the essential functions.

While performing the duties of this job, the employee is regularly required to stand; walk; use hands to probe, handle, or feel objects, tools, or controls; reach with hands and arms; and speak or hear. The employee is occasionally required to sit or stoop, kneel, or crouch.

The employee must regularly lift and/or move up to 100 pounds and frequently lift and/or move more than 100 pounds. Specific vision abilities required by this job include close vision, distance vision, peripheral vision, depth perception, and the ability to adjust focus.

**WORK ENVIRONMENT:** The work environment characteristics described here are representative of those an employee encounters while performing the essential functions of this job. Reasonable accommodations may be made to enable individuals with disabilities to perform the essential functions.

While performing the duties of this job, the employee is regularly exposed to bloodborne pathogens.

The noise level in the work environment is usually moderate.

rev. 9/95
rev. 6/96

**Figure 1-1** *(continued)*

experience, or willingness needed to complete an assignment, it is inappropriate to accept responsibility for an assignment.

Responsibility cannot be delegated if the assumption of the responsibility is not taken by the receiver of the assignment. Once a person accepts responsibility for an assignment, this responsibility is retained. For example, after the UAPs assigned duty is performed, the UAP is responsible to give feedback to the nurse about the performance and outcome of the duty. This

**TABLE 1-2**
*LEVELS OF AUTHORITY*

| Level | Authority |
|-------|-----------|
| One | Delegate to collect data to simply find out the facts or assess the situation and report back. |
| Two | Delegate to collect data and make a recommendation back to the RN. |
| Three | Delegate to assess the situation, make a recommendation, report back, and then implement the final RN recommendation. |
| Four | Delegate to carry out the task as they believe is appropriate. |

Adapted from Cox, SH, 1997. Motivation and Morale: Coin of the Realm. Symposium conducted at Nursing Management Congress.

feedback information is given in a specified time frame. Note that feedback works two ways. It is the UAP's responsibility to give feedback as well as the registered nurse's responsibility to follow up with ongoing supervision and evaluation of the UAP activities. The nurse transfers authority for the completion of a delegated task but retains responsibility and accountability for monitoring the delegated task's outcome.

## STOP AND THINK

A charge registered nurse assigned a new RN to start an IV line today. Yesterday, this charge nurse went with this same nurse to do the same procedure and noted that the new nurse was doing it properly. Today, the charge nurse asks the new nurse to do it alone. The new nurse says that she is comfortable doing it and will call the charge nurse if she needs help.
  Did the charge nurse delegate authority correctly?
  Did the new nurse correctly assume responsibility to do the IV?
  Who is accountable for the patient outcome?

## TYPES OF DELEGATION

There are two types of patient care activities that may be delegated; direct and indirect activities.

## Direct Patient Care Activities

Direct patient care activities include activities such as assisting the patient with feeding, drinking, ambulating, grooming, toileting, dressing, and socializing. Direct patient care activity may also involve reporting and documenting care related to these activities. These data are reported to the RN, who uses the information to make a clinical judgment about patient care. Activities delegated to UAP do not include health counseling or teaching or activities that require independent, specialized nursing knowledge, skill, or judgment.

**Nursing judgment** is defined as the process by which nurses come to understand the problems, issues, or concerns of clients, to attend to salient information, and to respond to client problems in concerned and involved ways (NCSBN, 1997). It includes both conscious decision-making and intuitive response.

## STOP AND THINK

It was just about 6:30 P.M. on the 3 P.M. to 11 P.M. shift on 2 East. Most of the physicians had made their rounds so the evening was calming down. The UAP, Jill, was picking up the dinner trays from the patient's rooms. Steve, the RN, had just sat down to document his patient assessments when he heard the UAP, Jill, yell "I need some help in Room 2510, Mr. Olson is not breathing." As several of the nurses ran to Room 2510, another UAP ran for the Emergency Crash Cart. The cart was wheeled into the patient's room during the overhead announcement by the operator, "CODE BLUE, Room 2510." The nurses initiated Cardio Pulmonary Resuscitation (CPR). The UAP plugged the cart into the wall, turned the suction machine on, and then assisted the family out of the room and stayed with them until the nurse was able to talk with them.

How does completion of these tasks by the UAP contribute to patient care? Does the UAP relieve the pressure on the nurse to complete everything? (See patient description, p. xxii)

## Indirect Patient Care Activities

**Indirect patient care** activities are often necessary to support the patients and their environment, and only incidentally involve direct patient contact. These activities are often designated "unit routines" and assist in providing a clean, efficient, and safe patient care milieu. They typically encompass chore services, companion care, housekeeping, transporting, clerical, stocking, and maintenance tasks (ANA, 1996).

## REAL WORLD INTERVIEW

If you think you don't want to use technicians and Certified Nursing Assistants (CNAs), you might want to sit down and make a list of all the duties they do. As the nursing population ages, do you want to push beds and stretchers, lift and turn heavy patients, assist patients in and out of their vehicles, and so forth? For myself, I have done team nursing and primary nursing and I definitely prefer to delegate!

The downside to delegation is that you may not always be familiar with the abilities of your technicians or CNAs. Appropriate patient care can't always be measured ahead of time with just a check-off sheet.

*Jan Robinson, RN, Austin, TX.*

## Underdelegation

Personnel in a new nursing role often underdelegate. Believing that older, more experienced staff may resent having someone new delegate to them, new nurses may simply avoid delegation. Or the new nurse may seek approval from other staff members by demonstrating their capability to complete all assigned duties without assistance.

New nurses can become frustrated and overwhelmed if they fail to delegate properly. They may also fail to delegate the appropriate authority to go with certain responsibilities. Perfectionism and refusal to allow mistakes can overwhelm a new nurse. More experienced staff members can help new personnel by intervening early and assisting in the delegation process, by clarifying roles and responsibilities, and by expressing willingness to work with the new RN.

## Overdelegation

Overdelegation of duties can also place the patient at risk. The reasons for overdelegation are numerous. Personnel may feel uncomfortable performing duties that are unfamiliar to them and they may depend too much on others. They may be unorganized or inclined to either avoid responsibility or immerse themselves in trivia. Overdelegation leads to delegating duties to personnel who are not educated for the tasks such as LPNs and UAP. Delegating duties that are inappropriate for personnel to perform because they have been inadequately educated is dangerous and against the state nurse practice act. Overdelegating duties can overwork some personnel and under-work others, creating obstacles to delegation. See Table 1-3.

**TABLE 1-3**
*OBSTACLES TO DELEGATION*

- Fear of being disliked.
- Inability to give up control of the situation.
- Inability to determine what to delegate and to whom.
- Past experience with delegation that did not turn out well.
- Lack of confidence to move beyond being a novice nurse.
- Tendency to isolate oneself and choosing to complete all tasks alone.
- Lack of confidence in delegating to staff that were previously one's peers.
- Inability to prioritize using Maslow's Hierarchy of Needs and the Nursing Process.
- Thinking of oneself as the only one who can complete a task the way it is supposed to be done.
- Inability to communicate effectively.
- Inability to develop working relationships with other team members.
- Lack of knowledge of the capabilities of staff including their competency, skill, experience, level of education, job description, and so on.

## STOP AND THINK

Mary, RN, was told by the UAP, Jill, that Mrs. Zurich, the patient in Room 2511, wanted something for pain. Then a physician approached Mary and wanted to know why he had not been called that morning regarding Mrs. Thomas, the patient in 2503, whose potassium level was 2.8 mEq/L. Then, nurse Colleen informed Mary that Mr. Clark, the patient in Room 2505 was also complaining of pain. Mary asked Colleen to tell him that she will be in to see him in a few minutes. She asked Colleen if she could reposition Mr. Clark for comfort in the meantime. Mary then went to check the patient in Room 2511. Was Mary's request to Colleen an appropriate request? Could Mary have had Jill help with anything?
(See patient description, p. xxii)

## ORGANIZATIONAL RESPONSIBILITY FOR DELEGATION

Certain elements must be in place in an organization in order for efficient nursing delegation to occur. These elements help assure nursing and medical quality. They also help clarify all health care staff's role within the organizational system. See Table 1-4.

**TABLE 1-4**
*ORGANIZATIONAL ELEMENTS NEEDED FOR EFFICIENT DELEGATION*

- Follow professional standards for education, licensure, and competency in all hiring decisions, orientation, and ongoing continuing education programs.
- Have clear job descriptions and ongoing licensing and credentialing policies for RNs, MDs, LPN/LVNs, UAP, and other health care staff. The organization must ensure that all staff are safe, competent practitioners before assigning them to patient care. Orient all staff to each other's roles and job descriptions.
- Facilitate clinical and educational specialty certification and credentialing of all practitioners and staff.
- Provide standards for ongoing supervision and periodic licensure/competency verification and evaluation of all staff.
- Provide access to professional health care standards, policies, procedures, library, and medication information with unit availability and efficient Internet access.
- Facilitate regular evidence-based review of critical standards, policies, and procedure.
- Have clear policies and procedures for delegation and chain of command reporting lines for all staff from RN to charge nurse to nurse manager to nurse executive and, as appropriate, to risk management, the hospital ethics committee, the chief executive officer, physicians, the chief of the medical staff, the board of directors, the State Licensing Board for Nursing and Medicine, and the Joint Commission on Accreditation of Health Care Organizations. See Figure 1-2 for an illustration of one such organizational chain of command.
- Provide administrative support for supervisors and staff who delegate, assign, monitor, and evaluate patient care.
- Clarify MD accountability, such as, if an MD delegates a nursing task to UAP, the MD is responsible for monitoring that care delivery. This must be spelled out in hospital policy. If the RN notes that the UAP is doing something incorrectly, the RN has a duty to intervene and to notify the ordering practitioner of the incident. The RN always has an independent responsibility to protect patient safety. Blindly relying on another nursing or medical practitioner is not permissible for the RN.
- Provide standards for regular RN evaluation of UAP and LPN/LVN and reinforce need for UAP and LPN/LVN accountability to RN. RNs must delegate and supervise. They cannot abdicate this professional responsibility.

*(continues)*

**Table 1-4** (*continued*)

- Develop physical, mental, and verbal "No Abuse" policies to be followed by all professional and nonprofessional health care staff. See literature application in Chapter 3.
- Consider applying for Magnet Status for your facility. This status is awarded by the American Nurses Credentialing Center to nursing departments that have worked to develop high quality nursing care, including the empowering of nursing decision-making and delegation in clinical practice. (http://www.nursingworld.org)
- Consider a shared governance model of nursing practice to empower nursing decision-making and delegation in clinical practice.
- Monitor patient outcomes, including nurse sensitive outcomes, staffing ratios, and other quality indicators, as well as developing ongoing clinical quality improvement practices.
- Maintain ongoing monitoring of incident reports, sentinel events, and other elements of risk management and performance improvement of the process and outcome of patient care.
- Develop systematic, error-proof systems for medication administration that ensure the Six Rights of medication administration: the right patient, right medication, right dose, right time, right route, and right documentation. Include computerized order entry.
- Provide documentation of routine maintenance for all patient care equipment.
- Attain JCAHO Patient Safety Goals, 2003.
- Develop safe patient transfer policies, intra-hospital and intra-agency.

Organizations fulfill their responsibility to staff and patients by developing these elements and defining a clear chain of command.

## Chain of Command

The RN, including the new graduate nurse, is accountable to the charge nurse and nurse manager of the unit. The nurse manager is accountable to the chief nursing executive, such as the vice president for nursing. The chief nursing executive is accountable to the chief executive officer. The hospital's chief executive officer is accountable to the board of directors. The board of directors is accountable to the community it serves and often to another larger hospital corporation, as well as to state nursing and medical licensing boards and to the Joint Commission on Accreditation of Healthcare Organizations (JCAHO). All are accountable for their actions to the patients and to the communities that they serve.

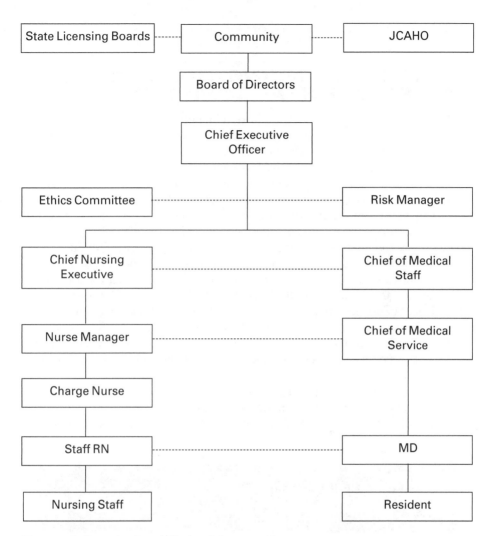

**Figure 1-2** Organizational Chain of Command

## STOP AND THINK

A novice RN was hired as a staff nurse. The nurse was assigned via the job description and nursing license to give nursing care to patients on the unit. When the nurse accepts this responsibility, the nurse is then accountable for the patient's care. May accountability be assigned to UAP?

    Why or why not?

    Is accountability shared with the charge nurse?

    Why or why not?

## CRITICAL THINKING, DECISION-MAKING, AND AN ETHICS TEST

The Pew Health Professions Commission identified that nurses must "demonstrate critical thinking, reflection, and problem solving skills" in order to thrive as effective practitioners in the Twenty-First century (Bellack & O'Neil, 2000). Paul (1992) defines **critical thinking** as "thinking about your thinking while you're thinking in order to make your thinking better" (p.7). A critical thinker is able to examine decisions from all sides and take into account varying points of view. A critical thinker does not say, "We've always done it this way," and refuse to consider alternate ways. The critical thinker generates new ideas and alternatives when making decisions. The critical thinker asks "why?" questions about a situation in order to arrive at the best decision. Four basic skills—critical reading, critical listening, critical writing, and critical speaking—are necessary for the development of critical thinking skills. These skills are developed as part of the process of developing and using thinking for decision-making. Ability in these four areas can be measured by the extent to which one uses the left side of the Universal Intellectual Standards as seen in Table 1-5. For example, a critical thinker works to be clear, precise, specific, accurate, and so on.

As you begin to apply critical thinking to nursing, use these Universal Intellectual Standards. Ask yourself whether the ideas are clear or unclear, precise or imprecise, specific or vague, accurate or inaccurate, and so forth.

| TABLE 1-5 | |
|---|---|
| *THE SPECTRUM OF UNIVERSAL INTELLECTUAL STANDARDS* | |
| Clear | Unclear |
| Precise | Imprecise |
| Specific | Vague |
| Accurate | Inaccurate |
| Relevant | Irrelevant |
| Consistent | Inconsistent |
| Logical | Illogical |
| Deep | Superficial |
| Complete | Incomplete |
| Significant | Insignificant |
| Adequate | Inadequate |
| Fair | Unfair |

Adapted from the foundation for critical thinking, Dillon, CA. http://criticalthinking.org/

Apply all of the Universal Intellectual Standards. You will improve your critical thinking skills, your decision-making skills, and your ability to delegate over time.

## Decision-Making Process and Delegation

While decisions to delegate patient care are unique to different situations, the decision-making process can be applied to each situation. There are five steps to the decision-making process. See Table 1-6.

Use of this five-step decision-making process will help the nurse make better decisions.

---

**TABLE 1-6**
*DECISION-MAKING PROCESS*

Five Steps of the Decision-Making Process.
- Identify the need for a decision.
- Determine the goal or outcome.
- Identify alternatives or actions with benefits and consequences of each.
- Choose an alternative.
- Evaluate the alternative chosen. Did you meet your goal?

From *Essentials of Leadership and Management,* Kelly-Heidenthal, 2004, p. 239.

---

# CASE STUDY

Apply the decision-making process.
1. Identify the need for a decision.
   You are caring for Mrs. Glusak, the patient in Room 2509 who recently had a CVA. Her husband is worried about her and asks you if he can stay tonight. Mrs. Glusak transferred from ICU two hours ago and is getting better.
2. Determine the goal or outcome.
   Your goal is to have both patient and wife maintain or improve their health. Mr. Glusak has told you that he has a heart condition himself. Staffing is good on the night shift.
3. Identify alternatives or actions with benefits and consequences of each.
   The alternatives are:
   A. Let him stay. The benefits are that he won't be worried. The consequences are that he may become exhausted over time.

*(continues)*

**Case Study** (*continued*)

    B. Talk with him and help him see the reasonableness of going home. The benefits are that he will get his rest. The consequences are that he may be thankful for the rest especially if you take the time to talk with him. He could also become annoyed at being encouraged to go home. Or he may talk you into letting him stay the night.

    C. Send him home with no discussion. Enforce the unit's "No visitors at night" policy. The benefit is that this may help him rest. The consequences are that he may become angry and worried and not rest. He may also think the hospital staff is unkind.

4. Choose an alternative.
    B was chosen.

5. Evaluate the alternative chosen. Did you meet your goal?
    After talking with him, he says he feels better and decides to go home. The next day he thanks you for taking the time to talk with him and tells you that he appreciated the rest, as well as the good care his wife is receiving.

(See patient desription, p. xxii)

# LITERATURE APPLICATION

**Citation:** Soukup, S. M. (2000). Preface to section on evidence-based nursing practice. *Nursing Clinics of North America, 35*(2), xvii–xviii.

**Discussion:** Author discusses a nurse's response to queries as to whether the nurse has integrated evidence-based practice. The nurse responds, "Yes, I practice state of the art nursing. My education and professional practice experiences have prepared me to care for more than 700 chronically ill patients annually in each of the past five years. These patients have an average reported expected pain rating of 6.9 (using a scale of 1 to 10, with 10 being severe pain). My pain management interventions have kept these patients, during my hours of care, at a reported actual pain rating of 4. Also, as a team member, these patients have not had any known pressure ulcers, skin tears, or catheter related infections. On two occasions, for patients that were dying, I created a humanizing environment for these patients and their families when they were rapidly transferred from the critical care unit. My documentation has met organizational standards during monthly peer reviews; I have provided leadership for emergencies with positive outcomes; and physician and patient satisfaction ratings for clinical practice on our unit is 9.5 on a scale of 10, with 10 being the highest. Our unit-based team has not had a needle stick related or back-related injury during the past two years. This has contributed to a significant cost avoidance and benefit to the organization."

(*continues*)

**Literature Application** (*continued*)

**Implications for Practice:** Nurses practicing in the twenty-first century must embrace the principles of evidence-based practice as an approach to effective decision-making, clinical care, and professional accountability.

# An Ethics Test

Health care practitioners may find that it is useful to run decision considerations through an ethics test when any doubt exists concerning an ethical issue. The ethics test presented here was used at the Center for Business Ethics at Bentley College (Bowditch & Buono, 1997) as part of ethical corporate training programs. Decision makers were taught to ask themselves:

- Is it right?
- Is it fair?
- Who gets hurt?
- Would you tell your child or young relative to do it?
- How does it smell? This question is based on a person's intuition and common sense.
- Would you be comfortable if the details of your decision were reported on the front page of your local newspaper or through your hospital's e-mail system?

# REVIEW QUESTIONS

1. Which of the following statements about RNs and UAP are true?
   A. UAP and RNs have equal responsibilities.
   B. UAP are responsible for all patient care.
   C. RNs are less accountable for patient care when UAP are assisting.
   D. RNs provide patient care delegating to other LPNs and UAP as necessary.

2. Which of the following is an inappropriate task for a LPN/LVN?
   A. Taking vital signs on a new patient.
   B. Completing a glucose Accucheck and reporting it to the RN.
   C. Completing a pain assessment that the UAP identified as being changed from an earlier assessment.
   D. Discharging a patient after teaching has been completed by the RN.

3. If a patient being discharged requires discharge nursing teaching, the most appropriate caregiver to perform this would be which of the following? The
   A. RN.
   B. LPN/LVN.
   C. MD.
   D. UAP.

 **REVIEW ACTIVITIES**

1. Read the study in the April 14, 1999, *Journal of the American Medical Association,* by Dr. Peter Pronovost and colleagues at the Johns Hopkins University. They found that a decreased ICU nurse-patient ratio during the day or evening was associated with increased ICU days and increased hospital length of stay. Could some of this high acuity patient care be safely delegated? Discuss.

2. Take an informal survey of UAP in the institution in which you are having your clinical practicum. Ask them what duties they are assigned. Ask them whether there are any duties with which they are not comfortable. Discuss your findings.

3. When you observe delegation of patient care on the unit, which of the obstacles identified in Table 1-3 have you noted? Have you seen the lack of knowledge of job descriptions interfere with delegation? Have you seen lack of confidence interfere with delegation? What else have you observed?

4. Identify a delegation problem that you have been considering. Using the decision-making grid at the bottom of this page, rate the alternative solutions to the problem that you have been considering on a scale of 1 to 3 on the elements of cost, quality, importance, and any other elements that are important to you.
   Did this exercise help you to clarify your thinking?

|  | Cost | Quality | Importance | Other |
|---|---|---|---|---|
| Alternative A |  |  |  |  |
| Alternative B |  |  |  |  |
| Alternative C |  |  |  |  |

# EXPLORING THE WEB

1. Check this site
   http://nclextestprep.com and click on the website for the state of Massachusetts identified there. Does your state have a similar site?

2. Logging on to Sigma Theta Tau International's website will access continuing education courses in leadership and management. Read the courses on delegation at this site.
   http://www.nursingsociety.org

3. Go to
   http://www.e-quipping.com/
   and click on delegation issues to view various views and issues on delegation.

4. Go to
   www.nursingworld.org
   and type in, nursing delegation, and note the information you find there.

5. Check this list of favorite healthcare websites

| | |
|---|---|
| http://www.aapcc.org | http://www.healthhelper.com |
| http://www.acb.org | http://www.health.discovery.com |
| http://www.acsh.org | http://www.healthy.net |
| http://www.ahrq.gov | http://www.intelihealth.com |
| http://www.allHealth.com | http://www.kidshealth.com |
| http://www.allnursingschools.com | http://www.lungusa.org |
| http://www.ama-assn.org | http://www.mayoclinic.com |
| http://www.americanheart.org | http://www.medlineplus.gov |
| http://www.arthritis.org | http://www.medscape.com |
| http://www.bestdoctors.com | http://www.ncsbn.org |
| http://www.cancer.org | http://www.netwellness.org |
| http://www.cdc.gov | http://www.ngc.gov |
| http://www.clinicaltrials.gov | http://www.nih.gov |
| http://www.cms.hhs.gov | http://www.nursingcenter.com |
| http://www.cochrane.org | http://www.nursingworld.org |
| http://www.diabetes.org | http://www.oncolink.org |
| http://www.drkoop.com | http://www.oxygen.com |
| http://www.eMD.com | http://www.pain.com |
| http://www.epilepsyfoundation.org | http://www.partnershipforcaring.org |
| http://www.familydoctor.org | http://www.pdr.net |
| http://www.fda.gov | http://www.personalMD.com |
| http://www.hcfa.gov | http://www.rarediseases.org |
| http://www.healthanswers.com | http://www.realage.com |
| http://www.healthAtoZ.com | http://www.rxlist.com |
| http://www.healthcentral.com | http://www.shapeup.org |
| http://www.healthfinder.gov | http://www.vh.org |
| http://www.healthgrades.com | http://www.webMD.com |

6. See a sample nurse practice act for practical nurses in Louisiana at http://www.lsbpne.com. How does this compare with this act in your state?

# REFERENCES

American Association of Critical Care Nurses (AACN). (1990). *Delegation of nursing and non-nursing activities in critical care: A framework for decision making.* Irvine, CA: AACN.

American Nurses Association (ANA). (1992). *Registered nurse utilization of unlicensed assistive personnel.* Washington, DC: American Nurses Publishing.

American Nurses Association (ANA). (1996). *Registered professional nurses and unlicensed assistive personnel* (2d ed.) Washington, DC: American Nurses Publishing.

American Nurses Association (ANA). (2001). Code of ethics for nurses with interpretive statements. Washington, DC: American Nurses Publishing.

Baggs, J. G., & Ryan, S. A. (1990). ICU nurse-physician collaboration and nursing satisfaction. *Nursing Economics, 8*(6), 386–392.

Barter, M., McLaughlin, F. E., & Thomas, S. A. (1997). Registered nurse role changes and satisfaction with unlicensed assistive personnel. *Journal of Nursing Administration, 27*(1), 29–38.

Bellack, J. P., & O'Neill, E. H. (2000). Recreating nursing practice for a new century: Recommendations and implications of the Pew Health Professions Commissions's final report. *Nursing and Health Care Perspectives, 21*(1), 14–21.

Benner, P. E. (2000). *From novice to expert: Excellence and power in clinical nursing practice (Commemorative Edition).* Upper Saddle River, NJ: Prentice Hall.

Bowditch, J. L., & Buono, A. F. (1996). A primer on organizational behavior. New York: Wiley.

Cardillo, D. W. (2001). *Your first year as a nurse.* Roseville, CA: Prima.

Cox, S. H. (1997, November). *Motivation and morale: Coin of the realm.* Symposium conducted at Nursing Management Congress.

Fisher, M. (2000, December). Do you have delegation savvy? *Nursing 2000, 30*(12), 58–59.

Franck, P., & Price, M. (1980). *Nursing management* (2nd Edition). New York, NY: NCSBN.

Hansten, R. I.; & Washburn, M. J. (1998). *Clinical delegation skills: A handbook for professional practice.* Gaithersburg, MD: Aspen Publications.

National Council of State Boards of Nursing (NCSBN). (1995). *Delegation concepts and decision-making process* (National Council Position Paper). Chicago, IL: Author.

National Council of State Boards of Nursing (NCSBN). (1997a). *Glossary-delegation Terminology.* Chicago, IL: Author.

National Council of State Boards of Nursing (NCSBN). (1997b). *The five rights of delegation.* Chicago, IL: Author.

Nightingale, F. (1859). Notes on nursing: What it is and what it is not. London: Harrison & Sons.

Paul, R. (1992). Critical thinking: What every person needs to survive in a rapidly changing world. Santa Rosa, CA: Foundation for Critical Thinking.

## SUGGESTED READINGS

Anthony, M. K., Standing, T., & Hertz, J. E. (2000). Factors influencing outcomes after delegation to unlicensed assistive personnel. *Journal of Nursing Administration,* (10), 474–481.

Fiesta, J. (1999, June). Informed consent: What health care professionals need to know, Part 1. *Nursing Management, 30*(6), 8–9.

Hansten, R. I., Washburn, M. J., & Kenyon, V. L. (1999). *Home care nursing delegation skills.* Frederick, MD: Aspen.

Parsons L. C. (1999). Building RN confidence for delegation decision-making skills in practice. *Journal of Nursing Staff Development, 15*(6), 263–269.

Walczak, M. B., & Absolon, P. L. (2001). Essentials for effective communication in oncology nursing: assertiveness, conflict management, delegation, and motivation. *Journal of Nursing Staff Development, 17*(3), 159–162.

Zimmermann, P. G. (1997, May). Delegating to unlicensed assistive personnel. *Nursing, 27*(5), 71.

# CHAPTER 2

# Delegation Decision-Making Grid and the Five Rights

## OBJECTIVES

*Upon completion of this chapter, the reader should be able to:*

1. Utilize the National Council of State Boards of Nursing Delegation Decision-Making Grid.
2. Describe the Five Rights of delegation.
3. Discuss the role of state boards of nursing in delegation.
4. Discuss sources of power.
5. Identify delegation responsibilities of health team members.
6. Review delegation suggestions for RNs.

*Helen Zurich, Room 2511, is a 78-year-old patient with diabetes mellitus and cellulitis of the right great toe. She is on bed rest and wants to get out of bed and walk around. She has been dizzy at times since her admission. To whom would you delegate her care? How would you retain responsibility and accountability for Helen's care delivery?*
(See patient description, p. xxii)

T he National Council of State Boards of Nursing (NCSBN) has developed a Decision-Making Grid for the nurse to use in delegating patient care. The grid evaluates such elements as the competency of the nurse and unlicensed assistive personnel (UAP) as well as the stability of the client in order to determine if client care can be delegated.

This chapter will discuss this grid, the role of state boards of nursing in delegation, delegation responsibilities of health team members, the Five Rights of delegation, sources of power, and other delegation suggestions for nurses.

## THE NATIONAL COUNCIL OF STATE BOARDS OF NURSING (NCSBN) DELEGATION DECISION-MAKING GRID

The NCSBN has developed a Delegation Decision-Making Grid with seven elements. Rating the seven elements on the grid assists the nurse in delivering care based on such considerations as the level of client stability and the competency of the UAP and the licensed nurse. A lower rating on the grid indicates that the activity can be safely delegated. A higher rating on the grid cautions one against delegation. For example, if the level of client stability is ranked a 3 (client condition is unstable or acute or has a strong potential for change) and the level of UAP competence is also rated a 3 (a novice in performing nursing care activities in the defined client population), that activity should probably not be delegated. Each of the seven grid elements is scored to assist in making the delegation decision. See Figure 2-1.

| Elements for Review | | client A | client B | client C | client D |
|---|---|---|---|---|---|
| **Activity/task** | **Describe activity/task:** | | | | |
| **Level of Client Stability** | **Score the client's level of stability:**<br>0. client condition is chronic/stable/predictable<br>1. client condition has minimal potential for change<br>2. client condition has moderate potential for change<br>3. client condition is unstable/acute/strong potential for change | | | | |
| **Level of UAP Competence** | **Score the UAP competence in completing delegated nursing care activities in the defined client population:**<br>0. UAP—expert in activities to be delegated, in defined population<br>1. UAP—experienced in activities to be delegated, in defined population<br>2. UAP—experienced in activities but not in population<br>3. UAP—novice in performing activities and in defined population | | | | |
| **Level of Licensed Nurse Competence** | **Score the licensed nurse's competence in relation to both knowledge of providing nursing care to a defined population and competence in implementation of the delegation process:**<br>0. Expert in the knowledge of nursing needs/activities of defined client population *and* expert in the delegation process<br>1. Either expert in knowledge of needs/ activities of defined client population and competent in delegation *or* experience in the needs/activities of defined client population and expert in the delegation process<br>2. Experienced in the knowledge of needs/activities of defined client population *and* competent in the delegation process<br>3. Either experienced in the knowledge of needs/activities of defined client population *or* competent in the delegation process<br>4. Novice in knowledge of defined population *and* novice in delegation | | | | |
| **Potential for Harm** | **Score the potential level of risk the nursing care activity has for the client (*risk is probability of suffering harm*):**<br>0. None<br>1. Low<br>2. Medium<br>3. High | | | | |
| **Frequency** | **Score based on how often the UAP has performed the specific nursing care activity:**<br>0. Performed at least daily<br>1. Performed at least weekly<br>2. Performed at least monthly<br>3. Performed less than monthly<br>4. Never performed | | | | |
| **Level of Decision-making** | **Score the decision-making needed, related to the specific nursing care activity, client (both cognitive and physical status) and client situation:**<br>0. Does not require decision making<br>1. Minimal level of decision making<br>2. Moderate level of decision making<br>3. High level of decision making | | | | |
| **Ability for Self Care** | **Score the client's level of assistance needed for self-care activities:**<br>0. No assistance<br>1. Limited assistance<br>2. Extensive assistance<br>3. Total care or constant attendance | | | | |
| | TOTAL SCORE | | | | |

**Figure 2-1** NCSBN Delegation Decision-Making Grid (Reprinted and used by permission of the National Council of State Boards of Nursing, copyright 1997.)

## REAL WORLD INTERVIEW

Each agency using the NCSBN Delegation Decision-Making Grid may want to adapt the grid as we have done, defining patient stability and the levels of potential for harm to avoid large differences in scores based on intuition or past experience of staff using the grid. See our revised grid in Figure 2-2. Also, the NCSBN grid does not incorporate the availability of the RN as an aspect for consideration, which could impact care and the RN's delegation decisions.

*Deloris Armstrong, RN, BSN, Senior Project Coordinator, Nursing Practice, SETON Medical Center of SETON Healthcare Network of Austin, Texas, Magnet Hospital*

## LITERATURE APPLICATION

**Citation:** Conger, M. M. (1999). Evaluation of an educational strategy for teaching delegation decision making to nursing students. *Journal of Nursing Education, 38*(9), 419–422.

**Discussion:** This article discusses the importance of incorporating learning experiences in delegation as an aspect of leadership experience for nursing students. The experience discussed included having the students use the Nursing Assessment Decision Grid. The students then reported what they learned in the clinical setting using their delegation decision-making skills.

**Implications for Practice:** Strategies for implementing delegation skills in the clinical setting are useful. The students discussed in this article are given an assignment of two patients. They rank the tasks associated with providing optimal care and then determine to whom the tasks should be delegated.

## THE FIVE RIGHTS OF DELEGATION

The NCSBN has spelled out Five Rights of delegation (NCSBN, 1997) that nurses may apply to their practice. These Five Rights are the right task, the right circumstance, the right person, the right direction and communication, and the right supervision. See the website for more Five Rights information at http://www.ncsbn.org. See Table 2-1.

| BNE | TASK/PROCEDURE | | | PATIENT | | UAP | | RN |
|---|---|---|---|---|---|---|---|---|
| | Safety of Task | Absence of Problem-Solving | Interactions of RN to Patient | Stability of Patient for Task Per RN Assessment | Predictability of Patient's Response to Task | Validation of Competency | Experience | Availability |
| C A T E | High chance of risk; difficult to treat  0 | Potential innovations which are not clearly defined  0 | Requires ongoing RN instruction throughout procedure  0 | Unstable, probable fluctuation if task is done  0 | Predictable negative response  0 | No validation of competency  0 | No experience with task or patient type  0 | Not available  0 |
| G O R I E S | Moderate chance of risk, treatable over time  1 | Options for innovations are clearly defined, but require a choice  1 | Require intermittent interactions by RN throughout procedure  1 | Currently stable, Possible fluctuation if task is done  1 | Response could be negative or positive  1 | Validation of competency: *Discretionary Deleg.* Org. approved educ. program  1 | Minimal experience with task and/or patient type  1 | Available by phone or in person over time  1 |
| O F | Low chance of risk; easily treatable, temporary  2 | Problem-solving has clearly defined option identified in procedure/ education  2 | RN interactions completed before and/or after procedure  2 | Stable, Fluctuations unlikely if task is done  2 | Minimal chance for negative response  2 | Validation of competency: *Discretionary Deleg.* Org. approved educ. program  2 | Recent or frequent experience with task and/or patient type  2 | Available; easy to find  2 |
| T A S K S | Minimal or no chance or risk; no treatment needed  3 | No innovations needed  3 | No RN interactions needed  3 | Consistently stable, No expected fluctuations if task is done  3 | Predictable favorable response  3 | *Most Commonly Deleg. Tasks* Competency validation per delegating RN  3 | Experience with specific task and patient  3 | Immediately available  3 |

SCALE

0 = Not Met
1 = Marginally Met
2 = Adequately Met
3 = Ideally Met

**Figure 2-2** SETON Healthcare Network, RN Critical-Thinking Grid for Delegation to UAP

The final decision for delegation is based upon the RN's professional judgement. (BNE 218.10.6)

Guidelines for Decision-Making

☐ If a "0" is selected for any of the criterion in any of the categories (RN, UAP, PATIENT, or TASK), it is recommended that the task *not* be delegated.
☐ If a "1" is selected in the RN or UAP categories, it is recommended that all criterion in the PATIENT and "TASK" categories be a "2" or "3".
☐ If a "1" is selected for any of the PATIENT or TASK categories, it is recommended that all criterion in the RN and UAP category be a "2" or "3".
☐ If a "2" or "3" is selected for each of the criterion in the PATIENT, TASK, RN, or UAP categories, the task may be delegated.
☐ Category "3" represents the ideal criterion for delegation.

Courtesy and used by permission of Joyce Batcheller, Senior vice president, chief nursing officer, Seton Healthcare Network, Austin, Texas.

## TABLE 2-1
### FIVE RIGHTS OF DELEGATION

| | |
|---|---|
| Right Task | • Has the agency established policies, procedures, and standards consistent with the state nurse practice act; federal, state and local regulations and guidelines for practice; nursing professional standards; and the ANA Code of Ethics (ANA, 2001)?<br>• Can this task be delegated to any staff?<br>• Are patient and community needs met? |
| Right Circumstance | • Are the setting and available resources conducive to safe care?<br>• Does staff understand how to do the task safely?<br>• Does the job description, education, and competency of the RN, LPN/LVN, and UAP match the patient requirements?<br>• Do staff carry out delegated tasks correctly?<br>• Do they have the resources, equipment, and supervision needed to work safely? |
| Right Person | • Is the right person delegating the right task to the right person to be performed on the right patient?<br>• Is the patient stable with predictable outcomes?<br>• Is it legally acceptable to delegate to this person?<br>• Do personnel have documented knowledge, skill, and competency to perform the task? |
| Right Direction/ Communication | • Does the RN communicate the task clearly with directions, specific steps of the task, limits, and expected outcomes?<br>• Are times for feedback specified?<br>• Is staff understanding of the task clarified?<br>• Can staff say, "I don't know how to do this and I need help," without jeopardizing their job? |
| Right Supervision | • Is there appropriate monitoring, intervention, evaluation, and feedback as needed?<br>• Does the RN answer staff questions and problem-solve as needed?<br>• Does the staff report task completion and patient response to the RN?<br>• Does the RN provide follow-up teaching and guidance to staff as appropriate?<br>• Are problems, particularly any sentinel events, clarified or reported via the chain of command and as needed to the state board of nursing and the Joint Commission on Accreditation of Health Care Organizations (JCAHO)? |

Adapted from National Council of State Boards of Nursing (NCSBN 1997). The Five Rights of Nursing.

## LITERATURE APPLICATION

**Citation:** Fisher, M. (2000). Do you have delegation savvy? *Nursing 2000, 30*(12), 58–59.

**Discussion:** This article outlines the Five Rights of delegation proposed by the National Council of State Boards of Nursing: the right task, right circumstance, right person, right direction and communication, and right supervision. Explicit examples of each are presented clearly. The author explains the authority behind delegation and who is directly responsible for the patient's care. A series of questions is used to determine if the task should be delegated. These include questions about the patient's stability, the UAP's competence and frequency with which the UAP has performed the specific task in the past, the competence of the nurse to make appropriate delegation decisions, the potential for harm, how much the patient is involved in care decisions, and what ability the patient has for self-care.

**Implications for practice:** The article is a good quick reference to review delegation and its implications.

## STATE BOARDS OF NURSING

Some states specify nursing tasks that may be delegated in their rules and regulations. The examples in Table 2-2 are similar to those of several states, but there is variation in rules and regulations from state to state. Check state requirements with your state board of nursing link at this website, http://www.ncsbn.org.

## KNOWLEDGE AND SKILL OF DELEGATION

Note that delegation is not a skill that is simply learned in a classroom. Delegation requires discussion of knowledge and concerns related to delegation and clinical mentorship or practice in responsibilities related to that delegation. The process also includes discussion of how to handle situations where tasks were not accomplished when delegated (Salmond, 1994).

## POWER

Nurses working in organizations use power when delegating patient care to others. Most researchers agree that sources of power and authority for nurses

**TABLE 2-2**

*DELEGATION TASK EXAMPLES*

Nursing Tasks That May *Not* Be Delegated
- Patient assessment (physical, psychological, and social assessment that requires professional nursing judgment, intervention, referral, or follow-up). Note that data collection without interpretation is not assessment.
- Planning of nursing care and evaluation of the patient's response to the care given.
- Implementation of patient care that requires judgment.
- Health teaching and health counseling other than reinforcement of what the RN has already taught.
- Medication Administration.

Tasks That Are Most Commonly Delegated
- Non-invasive and non-sterile treatments.
- Collecting, reporting, and documentation of data, such as
    ○ Vital signs, height, weight, intake and output, capillary blood and urine test for sugar, and hematest.
    ○ Ambulation, positioning, and turning.
    ○ Transportation of the patient within the facility.
    ○ Personal hygiene and elimination, including cleansing enemas.
    ○ Feeding, cutting up of food, or placing of meal trays.
    ○ Socialization activities.
    ○ Activities of daily living.

Nursing Tasks That May Not Be Routinely Delegated: Note that these may sometimes be delegated if the Staff has received special credentialing, such as education and competency testing.
- Sterile procedures.
- Invasive procedures, such as inserting tubes in a body cavity, or instilling or inserting substances into an indwelling tube.
- Care of broken skin other than minor abrasions or cuts generally classified as requiring only first aid treatment.

## LITERATURE APPLICATION

**Citation:** Johnson, S. H. (1996). Teaching nursing delegation: Analyzing nurse practice acts. *Journal of Continuing Education in Nursing, 27*(2), 52–58.

**Discussion:** This author notes the policies common to many state nurse practice acts. These policies include:
- Only nursing tasks can be delegated, not nursing practice.
- RN must perform patient assessment to determine what can be delegated.
- UAP do not practice professional nursing.
- RN can delegate only what is in the scope of nursing practice.
- LPN works under the direction/supervision of RN.
- RN delegates care based on the knowledge and skill of the person selected to perform the task.
- RN determines competency of the person to whom the nurse delegates.
- RN cannot delegate activity that requires RN professional skill and knowledge.
- RN is accountable and responsible for delegated tasks.
- RN must evaluate patient outcomes resulting from delegated activity.
- Health care facilities can develop special delegation protocols provided they meet state board of nursing delegation guidelines.
- Delegation requires critical thinking by the RN.

The author recommends reviewing your own state nurse practice act and looking for the following items to improve your own understanding of delegation:
- Definition of delegation
- Items that cannot be delegated
- Items that cannot be routinely delegated
- Guidelines for RN on what can be delegated
- Description of professional nursing practice
- Description of LPN/LVN and UAP roles
- Degree of supervision required
- Guidelines for lowering risk of delegation
- Warning about inappropriate delegation
- Restricted use of the word "nurse" to licensed nurses

**Implications for Practice:** Reviewing your own state's nurse practice act can increase your knowledge and skill in using delegation appropriately. Note that information about many state boards of nursing can be accessed at http://www.ncsbn.org.

Search this site for model nursing practice acts and then search the state boards of nursing link.

are diverse and vary from one situation to another. They also agree that sources of power are a combination of conscious and unconscious factors that allow an individual to influence others to do as that individual wants (Fisher & Koch, 1996). Articles and textbooks about nursing administration, educational leadership, and organizational management commonly include references to the work of Hersey, Blanchard, and Natemeyer (1979), which is an expansion of the power typology originally developed by French and Raven in 1959. This power typology helps nurses understand how different people perceive power and subsequently relate and delegate to others in the work setting to achieve patient care goals (Miller, 2003). Power is described as having a basis in expertise, legitimacy, reference (charisma), reward, coercion, or connection. More recently, information power and subordinate power have been added to these (Wells, 1998; Miller, 2003; DuBrin, 2000). Generally speaking, nurses exert influence derived from one power source or a combination of power sources. See Table 2-3.

The way that power is used to delegate or accomplish a goal often determines its desirability and how others perceive it. Effective nurses use sources of power, as appropriate, when delegating care. They combine referent (charismatic) power and expert power from a legitimate power base, adding carefully measured portions of reward power and little or preferably no coercive power. These nurses gather and use information in new and creative ways. They understand that power should be a means to accomplish a goal instead of a goal in itself. Effective nurses also recognize that power is earned and that power should not be defined merely as bad or good (Strasen, 1987). Understanding and using these sources of power assists the nurse when delegating care.

Ultimately, some professional activities involving the specialized knowledge, judgment, or skill of the nursing process can never be delegated. These include patient assessment, triage, making a nursing diagnosis, establishing nursing plans of care, extensive teaching or counseling, telephone advice, evaluating outcomes, and discharging patients (Zimmermann, 1996). Delegated tasks are typically those tasks that occur frequently, are considered technical by nature, are considered standard and unchanging, have predictable results, and have minimal potential for risks (Westfall, 1998). As a professional standard for all nurses in all states, the assessment, analysis, diagnosis, planning, teaching, and evaluation stages of the nursing process may not be delegated. Delegated activities usually fall within the implementation phase of the nursing process.

**TABLE 2-3**

*SOURCES OF POWER*

| Sources of Power | How Power Works |
|---|---|
| Expert Power (Fisher & Koch, 1996) | Expert power comes from the knowledge and skills that nurses possess. The greater any nurse's proficiency in performing his or her role, the greater is the nurse's expert power. This power should be acknowledged by others to be most effective. |
| Legitimate Power (Fisher & Koch, 1996) | Legitimate power is derived from the position a nurse holds in a group, and it indicates the nurse's degree of authority. Legitimate power is based on such factors as licensure, academic degrees, certification, experience in the role, and title/position in the institution. |
| Referent (Charisma) Power (Fisher & Koch, 1996) | Referent power is derived from the admiration, trust, and respect that people feel toward an individual, group, or organization. The referent person has the ability to inspire confidence. In any situation, strong referent leaders are considered charismatic and people of great vision, which may or may not be the reality. |
| Reward or Coercion Power (Miller, 2003) | The ability to reward or punish others as well as the power to create fear in others to influence them to change their behavior is commonly termed reward power or coercive power. |
| Connection Power (Miller, 2003) | Both personal and professional relationships are part of a nurse's connections. People who are strongly connected to others, both personally and professionally, have enhanced resources and enhanced capacity for learning and sharing information. They have a broader overall sphere of influence. Teamwork, collaboration, networking, and mentoring are some of the ways that a nurse can become more connected and therefore more powerful. See Table 2-4. |

*(continues)*

**Table 2-3** (*continued*)

| | |
|---|---|
| Information Power (Miller, 2003) | Information power is power based on the information that any person can provide to the group. Authoritarian leaders attempt to control information. Charismatic leaders provide information that is seductive for many people. Information leaders provide a sense of stability with the use and synthesis of information. If one knows how to obtain information, and what to do with it, some believe the greatest power may be in information. |
| Subordinate Power (DuBrin, 2000) | Subordinate power is any type of power that employees can exert upward in their organization based on legal and justice considerations. When subordinates perceive an order as being outside the limits of legitimate authority, they have the power to rebel. |

Adapted from Miller, T. in Kelly-Heidenthal, P. L., Nursing Leadership & Management, 2003, Delmar.

## STOP AND THINK

What type of power have you observed on the clinical unit? Have you seen power used by RNs, MDs, and UAP? How can nurses improve their use of power in delegating patient care? Where does nursing power come from?

# DELEGATION RESPONSIBILITIES OF HEALTH TEAM MEMBERS

A new graduate nurse may feel overwhelmed in his or her first nursing position by the responsibility of patient care, especially if patient needs are urgent. New graduate nurses may quickly realize that if they do not delegate some of the patient's care, it will not be completed in a timely and effective manner. Other staff can help the new graduates with this and help them develop their roles and teach them how to delegate. Other staff can also help by introducing department staff and explaining their roles to the new nurses.

## Nurse Manager Responsibility

The nurse manager helps develop staff members' ability to delegate. Guidance in this area is necessary because new graduates, wanting to be regarded favorably, often try to do everything themselves and do not ask for assistance.

**TABLE 2-4**

*WASHINGTON'S MOST POWERFUL LOBBYING GROUPS*

1. National Rifle Association
2. American Association of Retired Persons
3. National Federation of Independent Business
4. American Israel Public Affairs Committee
5. Association of Trial Lawyers
6. AFL-CIO
7. Chamber of Commerce
8. National Beer Wholesalers Association
9. National Association of Realtors
10. National Association of Manufacturers
11. National Association of Home Builders
12. American Medical Association
13. American Hospital Association
14. National Education Association
15. American Farm Bureau Federation

From "Fat & Happy in D.C.," *Fortune,* May 28, 2001, p. 95.

Orientation will cover staff job descriptions, competency, chain of command guidelines, and other organizational resources for the new nurse. Delegation is a skill that will require much guidance and practice.

The nurse manager will determine the appropriate mix of personnel on a nursing unit based on the patient's needs, acuity level, and staff competency. From this personnel mix, the nurse manager will identify who can best perform the direct and indirect nursing duties. This information is shared with new nurses to assist in determining appropriate delegation.

# New Graduate Registered Nurse Responsibility

New graduate registered nurses need to focus on the duties for which they are directly responsible. What duties can they delegate and to what extent? What do UAP do? What do licensed practical nurses/licensed vocational nurses (LPNs/LVNs) do? The state nurse practice act and the job description of each of these staff will help clarify the responsibilities of each staff member.

# Registered Nurse Responsibility

The registered nurse is responsible and accountable for the provision of nursing care. Although UAP may measure vital signs, intake and output, and other patient status indicators, it is the registered nurse who analyzes this data for comprehensive assessment, nursing diagnosis, implementation, and evaluation of the plan of care. The RN also remains responsible for the patient outcome.

## REAL WORLD INTERVIEW

I use delegation now that I have completed school. I began working as a graduate nurse immediately after graduating nursing school. Prior to graduation, I worked as a nurse technician. I feel that I understand how it feels to be at both ends of patient care delivery. I vowed that when I became a registered nurse, I would delegate appropriately and fairly to others.

As a registered nurse I make a point to delegate appropriately to certified nursing assistants (CNAs). I delegate duties like vital signs, changing beds, bathing patients, feeding patients, and performing accurate intake and output. I delegate these things after giving my CNA a complete report of my patients.

I work on a medical-surgical floor where our CNAs use an automated DYNAMAP vital sign monitor to take blood pressures, pulses, and temperatures. I will take a manual blood pressure when I am assessing my patient if the automated readings from the DYNAMAP monitor are high or low. My CNAs bring me their vital signs as soon as they are done, so that I can determine what more I need to evaluate.

It is important to mention that I never delegate patient assessments or patient education. These duties are reserved for the registered nurse. I will never delegate a CNA to watch over patients while they take their medication. I never delegate the insertion or removal of Foleys. I do believe my CNAs take me seriously as I do not delegate anything that I am not willing to do myself and have not done myself in the past. In essence, I do not give the impression that I am "beyond" or "better" than anyone else.

I get concerned when I see a fellow nurse walk out of a patient's room who has just requested a bedpan and goes to find a CNA to get him that bedpan. I would never make my patient wait to perform such a necessary task. As I said earlier, I have been on both ends of patient care delivery and I know how it feels to be unappreciated. So far, I have stuck to my promise to delegate appropriately and fairly. I truly believe my CNAs would agree.

*Shelly A. Thompson, new graduate nurse*

# Licensed Practical/Vocational Nurse (LPN/LVN) Responsibility

LPN/LVN caregivers who have undergone a standardized training and competency evaluation are able to perform duties and functions that UAP are not allowed to do. LPN/LVNs are held to a higher standard of care and are responsible for their actions. Common LPN/LVN duties include the duties of the

UAP as well as reinforcing teaching from a standard care plan and updating initial assessments. In many states, with documented competency, LPN/LVN duties may also include initiating and/or maintaining intravenous lines, blood transfusions, and hyperalimentation lines, giving IV push and piggy back medications, inserting feeding tubes, and so on. The LPN works under the direction of the RN and their roles must be in agreement with the state nurse practice act and should be reflected in policies, job descriptions, methods of assigning, and competency documentation, no matter what the setting. See a sample scope of practice for practical nurses in Louisiana at http://www.lsbpne.com. Search for scope of practice.

The RN must be aware of the job description, skills, and educational background of the LPN/LVN prior to delegation of duties. Note that the RN is still primarily responsible and accountable for overall patient assessment, planning, implementation and evaluation of the quality of care delegated to the LPN/LVN. See Figure 2-3.

## STOP AND THINK

Identify a group of four patients on the unit where you have your clinical experience. Note the RNs, LPN/LVNs, and UAP on the unit. Practice delegation decision-making using the Five Rights of delegation and the NCSBN Delegation Decision-Making Grid with this group of patients and staff. How did it go? What issues did you have to work out? Would you make the same delegation decision again?

## REAL WORLD INTERVIEW

Upon evaluating delegation over the course of several, varied nursing units, I arrived at one conclusion: we as professional nurses just do not do it well. There is the exception, of course, that being the individual who has developed an outstanding ability to delegate nearly all of his or her responsibilities to others in an authoritative or diplomatic manner with the recipients either loving or hating it.

I tend to believe that part of the problem lies with the job description, that black-and-white document that delineates the role in great detail right up to the final statement of "inclusive of duties as assigned." Duties as assigned leads one to think that someone will be assigning something, to someone. It is too vague and I just hope that the delegated task is clearly stated somewhere in someone's job description.

*(continues)*

**Real World Interview** (*continued*)

On a nursing unit, it generally falls on the charge nurse to function in the assigning and delegating role. For this role, he or she is often criticized, most frequently behind the scenes, though occasionally he or she is blasted right out in the open. "What do you mean I am getting the next admission? I already have gotten two!" At best, one becomes apprehensive when assigning anything, from an admission to cleaning up the break room. I wonder, if that is the fate of the charge nurse, just how well would one expect the staff RN to delegate?

Perhaps our failures with delegation stem from our predominately female, motherly, gender. Moms can do it! Moms can do it all. Often, Mom finds the route of least resistance: "It's just easier to do it myself!" It is the same thing with RNs; RNs can do it, RNs can do it all.

I believe that the fine art of delegation needs to be taught more in the educational process, along with the concept of teamwork. The team is hindered when we become ineffective at delegation. The challenges of contemporary health care are tremendous and will only become more challenging in the future. We as professional nurses would do well to acquire advanced skills in delegation, teambuilding, and diplomacy for these skills will become tools of survival in the very near future.

*Suzanne Kalweit,* RN, MS

# Unlicensed Assistive Personnel (UAP) Responsibility

The increased numbers of UAP in acute care settings pose a degree of risk to the patient. The House of Representatives Patient Safety Act of 1996 assists in the campaign for safe staffing levels using an appropriate skill mix for patient outcomes. The Act assures that every patient is assigned a registered nurse. According to the Act, UAP may perform duties such as bathing, feeding, toileting, and ambulating patients. UAP also report information related to these activities. The RN will delegate to the UAP and is liable for those delegations. According to the ANA (1992), if the RN knows or reasonably believes that the assistant has the appropriate training, orientation, and documented competencies, then the RN can reasonably expect that the UAP will function in a safe and effective manner.

Using UAP in acute care settings frees RNs from non-nursing duties and allows time for RNs to complete assessments of patients and their responses to treatments. It is less expensive to have UAP perform non-nursing duties than

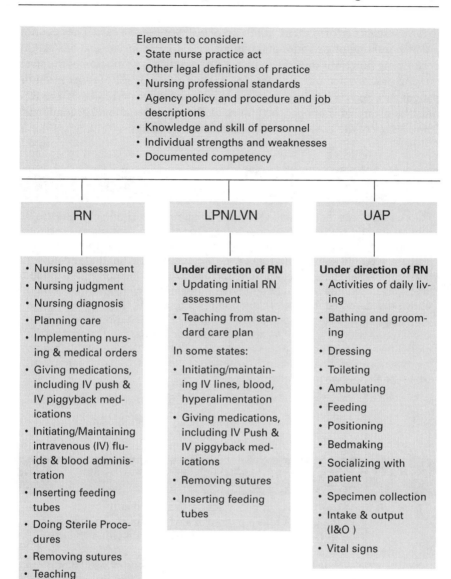

Elements to consider:
• State nurse practice act
• Other legal definitions of practice
• Nursing professional standards
• Agency policy and procedure and job descriptions
• Knowledge and skill of personnel
• Individual strengths and weaknesses
• Documented competency

### RN

• Nursing assessment
• Nursing judgment
• Nursing diagnosis
• Planning care
• Implementing nursing & medical orders
• Giving medications, including IV push & IV piggyback medications
• Initiating/Maintaining intravenous (IV) fluids & blood administration
• Inserting feeding tubes
• Doing Sterile Procedures
• Removing sutures
• Teaching
• Evaluation

### LPN/LVN

**Under direction of RN**
• Updating initial RN assessment
• Teaching from standard care plan

In some states:
• Initiating/maintaining IV lines, blood, hyperalimentation
• Giving medications, including IV Push & IV piggyback medications
• Removing sutures
• Inserting feeding tubes

### UAP

**Under direction of RN**
• Activities of daily living
• Bathing and grooming
• Dressing
• Toileting
• Ambulating
• Feeding
• Positioning
• Bedmaking
• Socializing with patient
• Specimen collection
• Intake & output (I&O )
• Vital signs

**Figure 2-3** Considerations in Delegation

to have nurses perform them. UAP can deliver supportive care. They cannot practice nursing or provide total patient care. Inappropriate use of UAP in performing functions outside their scope of practice is a violation of the state nursing practice act and is a threat to patient safety. The RN must monitor patient care and patient outcomes when tasks are delegated to UAP. The RN must be aware of the job description, skills, educational background, and competency of the UAP prior to the delegation of duties.

## REAL WORLD INTERVIEW

I work as a nurse technician I at a local hospital. I was sitting at the nurse's station after finishing my afternoon vitals. One of the nurses approached me saying that she was really busy and she was getting an admission. She handed me an IV solution and asked me to hang it. I told her that I could not do it. She replied to me that it was no big deal and that I was almost a nurse. She walked away saying that it should be hung at 100 cc/hr. Being concerned about my career that I hadn't even started to practice, I did not do it. I approached the charge nurse and told her my situation. Knowing that the other nurse was busy, she checked the medication sheets and hung the infusion. She approached the other nurse about the situation and explained to her that it was wrong to ask me to do what she did, and to put me in that position. The first nurse just walked away.

*Jill Conner, Nurse Technician*

## STOP AND THINK

These are some examples of appropriate delegation of authority:
- An RN asks the UAP to take a patient in a wheelchair for a chest x-ray.
- The charge nurse asks another RN to be in charge while she goes to dinner.
- The RN asks the LPN to reinforce the teaching of the low salt diet when the lunch trays come.

Why are these delegations appropriate?

Why must the nurse evaluate staff qualifications, skill, job description, competency, and patient need prior to delegation?

Are there times when these delegation examples may not be safely delegated?

# LITERATURE APPLICATION

**Citation:** Sheehan, J. P. (2001). Delegating to UAP—A practical guide. *RN,* *64*(11), 65–66.

**Discussion:** Delegating duties to unlicensed assistive personnel can free up the RN to complete RN level tasks. To do this without endangering patients or increasing the RN's liability, the RN should consider the key questions this article discusses:

What should you do before you delegate? What can you delegate and what can't you delegate? How should you effectively assign tasks? How can you minimize your liability?

**Implications for Practice:** Specific delegation scenarios are discussed in this article. The National Council of State Boards of Nursing Five Rights of delegation is discussed and the examples are useful for nurses to improve their ability to delegate in various situations.

# DELEGATION SUGGESTIONS FOR RNS

RNs concerned with appropriate delegation find it helpful to use the delegation suggestions in Table 2-5.

**TABLE 2-5**

*DELEGATION SUGGESTIONS FOR RNS*

- Consider prior to delegating
    - Who has the time to complete the delegated project?
    - Who is the best person for the project?
    - What is the urgency of the project?
    - Are there any deadlines?
    - Which staff need to develop their skills?
    - Which staff would enjoy the project?

- Be clear on the qualifications of the delegate, such as education, experience, and competency. Require documentation or demonstration of current competence by the delegate for each task. Clarify patient care concerns or delegation problems. Click on ANA position statements at http://www.nursingworld.org and your state board of nursing, as necessary.

*(continues)*

**Table 2-5** (*continued*)

- Speak to your delegates as you would like to be spoken to. There is no need to apologize for your delegation. Remember, you are carrying out your professional responsibility.

- Communicate the patient's name, room number, and duty to be performed. Identify the timeframe for completion. Discuss any changes from the usual procedures that might be needed to meet special patient needs and any potential patient abnormalities that should be reported to the RN. The expectations for personnel before, during, and after duty performance should be stated in a clear, pleasant, direct, and concise manner.

- Identify the expected patient outcome and the limits of the delegate's authority.

- Verify the delegate's understanding of delegated tasks and have the delegate repeat instructions, as needed. Verify that the delegate accepts responsibility and accountability for carrying out the task correctly. Require frequent mini-reports about patients from staff.

- Avoid removing duties once assigned. This should be considered only when the duty is above the level of the personnel as when the patient's care is in jeopardy because the patient's status has changed.

- Monitor task completion according to standards. Make frequent walking rounds to assess patient outcomes.

- Accept minor variations in the style in which the duties are performed. Individual styles are acceptable if the standards are met and good outcomes are achieved.

- Try to meet staff needs for learning opportunities and consider any health problems and work preferences of the staff as long as it doesn't interfere with meeting patient needs.

- If a delegate doesn't meet the standards, talk with him or her to identify the problem. If this is not successful, inform the delegate that you will be discussing the problem with your supervisor. Document your concerns, as appropriate. Follow up with your supervisor according to your organization's policy.

Adapted from Boucher, MA 1998. Delegation Alert. American Journal of Nursing, 98(2), 26–32, and Zimmerman, PG (1996, June). Delegating to Assistive Personnel. Journal of Emergency Nursing, 22(3), 206–212.

## CASE STUDY

Practice filling out the NCSBN Delegation Decision-Making Grid in Figure 2-1 with the core list of patients at the front of this textbook. Identify what the patients' needs are and identify what you can safely delegate. Remember, the lower the score on the Grid, the more likely the care can be delegated. Identify sample staff that you can use in this case study from one of your clinical units.

## REVIEW QUESTIONS

1. When a person or a group fears another enough to act or behave differently than otherwise, the source of power is called:
   A. Coercive power
   B. Reward power
   C. Expert power
   D. Connection power

DISCARDED

2. What source of power has become increasingly important because of technological innovation through the last decade?
   A. Expert power
   B. Information power
   C. Connection power
   D. Legitimate power

3. A new graduate nurse asks the charge nurse, "How do I know what I can and cannot delegate?" What is the best reply the charge nurse can give in this situation?
   A. "You will not be delegating, only the charge nurse delegates, so there is nothing to worry about."
   B. "You can work it out with your UAP."
   C. "Delegate the tasks that you don't have time for so all the work gets done."
   D. "The state we work in has a nurse practice act to guide you."

4. When the nurse considers delegating a task, what Five Rights should be considered?
   A. Right task, right circumstance, right person, right direction/communication, right supervision
   B. Right route, right time, right patient, right documentation, right dose
   C. Right patient, right chart, right physician, right results, right information
   D. Right supervision, right patient, right task, right documentation, right time frame

5. The charge nurse working with an RN, an LPN, and a UAP is very busy with the group of patients on the unit. One patient's intravenous line has just infiltrated, a physician is on the phone waiting for a nurse's response, a patient wants to be discharged, and the UAP has just reported an elevated temperature on a new surgical patient. Who should be assigned to restart the intravenous line? The
   A. LPN
   B. UAP
   C. RN
   D. Charge nurse

6. Which patient will you delegate to the LPN?
   A. The patient who has a fleet enema ordered.
   B. The patient who needs to be started on a 24-hour urine collection.
   C. The patient who is elderly and needs help with frequent ambulation.
   D. The patient who is two days post-op and needs an abdominal wound irrigation and dressing change every shift.

## ■ REVIEW ACTIVITIES

1. You are caring for a new patient in Room 2510. You are trying to decide whether to delegate his care to UAP Jill or to UAP Penny. Use the Decision-Making Grid in Table 2-6 to decide.

**TABLE 2-6**
***DECISION-MAKING GRID***

|  | Certified? | Easy to work with? | Do their fair share? | Other? |
|---|---|---|---|---|
| Jill |  |  |  |  |
| Penny |  |  |  |  |

2. Have you had any clinical opportunities to delegate duties? Identify to whom and what you delegated and discuss how it affected the patient and your work. What would you do next time? Would you do anything differently? Was patient safety affected?

# EXPLORING THE WEB

Which sites can you visit for information on power and nurses?
http://google.com. Search for "nurse power."

What has a funny, not scholarly, synopsis of nursing power?
http://www.NursingPower.net

# REFERENCES

American Nurses Association. *Code of ethics for nurses with interpretive statements* (2001). Washington, DC: American Nurses Publishing.

American Nurses Association. *Registered nurse utilization of unlicensed assistive personnel* (1992). Washington, DC: American Nurses Publishing.

Battaglia, C. (1996). *Murmurs.* Long Branch, NJ: Vista.

Boucher, M. A. (1998). Delegation alert. *American Journal of Nursing, 98*(2), 26–32.

Conger, M. M. (1999). Evaluation of an educational strategy for teaching delegation decision making to nursing students. *Journal of Nursing Education, 38*(9), 419–422.

DuBrin, A. J. (2000). *The Active Manager* (5th ed.). South-Western College Publishing. London: International Thomson Publishing.

Fisher, M. (2000). Do you have the delegation savvy? *Nursing 2000, 30*(12), 58–59.

Fisher, J. L., & Koch, J. V. (1996). *Presidential leadership: Making a difference.* Phoenix, AZ: American Council on Education and The Oryx Press.

Hersey, P., Blanchard, K., & Natemeyer, W. (1979). Situational leadership, perception and impact of power. *Group and Organizational Studies, 4,* 418–428.

Johnson, S. H. (1996). Teaching nursing delegation: Analyzing nurse practice acts. *Journal of Continuing Education in Nursing, 27*(2), 52–58.

Miller, T. (2003). Power. In P. Kelly-Heidenthal (Ed.), *Nursing leadership and management.* Clifton Park, NY: Thomson Delmar Learning.

National Council of State Boards of Nursing. (1997). *The five rights of delegation.* Chicago, IL: Author.

Salmond, S. (1994). *Perceived effectiveness of models of care using clinical nursing assistants.* Pitman, NJ: National Association of Orthopedic Nurses.

Strasen, L. (1987). *Key business skills for nurse managers.* Philadelphia: J.B. Lippincott.

Sheehan, J. P. (2001). Delegating to UAPs—A practical guide. *RN, 64*(11), 65–66.

Wells, S. (1998). *Choosing the future: The power of strategic thinking.* Boston: Butterworth-Heinemann.

Zimmerman, P. G. (1996). Delegating to assistive personnel. *Journal of Emergency Nursing, 22*(3), 206–212.

## SUGGESTED READINGS

Baker, C., Beglinger, J., King, S., Salyards, M., & Thompson, A. (2000). Transforming negative work cultures. *Journal of Nursing Administration, 30*(7/8), 357–363.

Castledine, G. (2002). Prioritizing care is an essential nursing skill. *British Journal of Nursing, 11*(14), 987.

Fiesta, J. (1999). Informed consent: What health care professionals need to know, Part 1. *Nursing Management, 30,* 8–9.

Jervis, L. L. (2002). Working in and around the "chain of command": Power relations among nursing staff in an urban nursing home. *Nursing Inquiry, 9*(1), 12–23.

Moll, J. A., & Tripp, E. (2002). Nursing delegation: Implications for home care. *Caring, 21*(9), 24–28, 30, 32.

Sieloff, C. L. (2003). Measuring nursing power within organizations. *Journal of Nursing Scholarship, 35*(2), 183–187.

# CHAPTER 3

"Fundamentally who we are and how we work together is what our patients receive." (Nancy Moore, 2000)

# Effective Communication

## OBJECTIVES

*Upon completion of this chapter, the reader should be able to:*

1. Identify elements of the communication process.

2. Discuss the use of communication skills in delegation.

3. Discuss the impact of culture on delegation.

4. Review the professional role of the nurse.

5. Review potential barriers to communication.

6. Discuss helpful and non-helpful roles in communication.

7. Identify Myers-Briggs Personality Types.

8. Discuss workplace communication, including communicating with superiors and other practitioners.

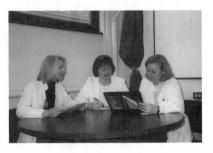

*As a newly licensed RN working in an adult unit in your agency, you begin your shift by making rounds on your patients to perform initial assessments. You enter Room 2501, Mr. Zagone, who has a long history of HIV. He was admitted last night with pneumonia. He is well known to the experienced staff. As you assess his breath sounds, he tells you with eyes downcast, "I don't think I'm going to make it this time." His wife, who is at his bedside, replies "Don't talk like that."*

*What are your thoughts about this situation?*

*What nonverbal cues might be used to help you interpret this message?*

*What communication skills will you use to respond appropriately?*

*How can you and your staff demonstrate caring behavior to Mr. Zagone and his wife?*

(See patient description, p. xxi)

Today's nurses use basic principles of communication to promote smooth interactions with patients, family members, nursing peers, and other disciplines. These communication principles allow nurses to adapt to trends that impact the profession of nursing and its practice. Additionally, nurses use communication skills to effectively delegate patient care to others. This chapter will discuss elements of the communication process, the impact of culture on delegation, potential barriers to communication, the Myers-Briggs Personality Types, and workplace communication. It will review the professional role of the nurse.

# ELEMENTS OF THE COMMUNICATION PROCESS

**Communication** is the sending and receiving of a message. Communication has six elements. These elements include sender, message, communication channel, receiver, feedback, and educational, cultural, emotional, and perceptual influences (White & Duncan, 2002). See Figure 3-1.

## Sender and Message

A message originates with the sender. Lasswell's classic model of Communication (1948) describes the sender as the "who" in communication. If the nurse initiates communication, the nurse is the sender. The message originates with the sender. It consists of verbal and/or nonverbal stimuli that are taken in by the receiver.

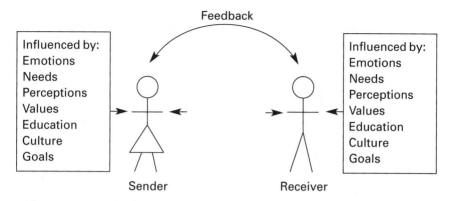

**Figure 3-1** Communication Process. (White, L and Duncan, G, Medical Surgical Nursing, 2002, Delmar, Albany, NY).

# Communication Channel and Receiver

The communication channel used by the sender to send the message may be verbal or nonverbal. The receiver takes in the message and analyzes it. When the nurse listens to a patient-initiated conversation, the nurse is the receiver. When the nurse receiver reacts by returning a new message to the patient, the receiver and sender reverse roles.

# Feedback and Educational, Cultural, Emotional, and Perceptual Influences

The new message that is generated by the receiver in response to the original message from the sender is the feedback. Bradley & Edinberg (1986) describe feedback as the "with what effect" and note that feedback is effective when the two communicators are sensitive to each other's messages and they change behaviors based on the message exchanges. Both the sender and the receiver are influenced by their education, culture, emotions, perceptions, goals, needs, values, and by the situation in which they find themselves.

# COMMUNICATION AND DELEGATION

Communication is a cornerstone to achieving success when delegating patient care. Optimal patient outcomes are achieved when the initial directions of the nurse clearly define the expectations of the unlicensed assistive personnel (UAP) or Licensed Practical Nurse/Licensed Vocational Nurse (LPN/LVN) in performing the assigned task. The use of the "Four Cs" in giving initial directions can help improve the communication of delegated tasks. (Zerwekh and Claborn, 2002). See Table 3-1.

A common pitfall when working with individuals for long periods of time is that people fall into routines. When this happens, less talking may occur and unrealistic expectations can occur. This can be positive or negative for the patient. The Joint Commission on Accreditation of Healthcare Organizations (JCAHO) announced National Patient Safety Goals for 2003. Included in the goals are recommendations on improving the effectiveness of communication among caregivers.

http://www.jcaho.org  Click on Patient Safety Goals.

The main reason for effective communication is clear. Safe, quality patient care is compromised when lack of communication occurs among those providing care. Examples such as "I thought you said . . ." or "Didn't I ask you to let me know how the procedure went?" or "Well, that's isn't what I meant . . ." not to mention "Nobody ever told me to do it that way . . . are classic examples of comments people make when communication problems occur.

## Communication Skills

Effective communication requires that both parties use communication skills that enhance a particular interaction. Baker, Beglinger, King, Salyards and Thompson (2000) believe that the most important considerations to facilitate communication are to be open and willing to give and receive feedback. Some of the most important skills nurses rely on to facilitate communication are attending, responding, clarifying, and confronting skills.

| TABLE 3-1 | |
| :--- | :--- |
| *FOUR C'S OF COMMUNICATION* | |
| CLEAR | Does the team member understand what I am saying? |
| CONCISE | Have I confused the direction by giving too much unnecessary information? |
| CORRECT | Is the direction given according to policy, procedure, job description, and the law? |
| COMPLETE | Does the delegate have all the information necessary to complete the task? |

Adapted from Zerwekh, J., and Claborn, J., 2002. Nursing Today: Transition and Trends. St. Louis, Missouri. Saunders.

# REAL WORLD INTERVIEW

I view my primary responsibility as a nurse to be that of patient advocate. As a team leader, I am responsible for coordinating patient care for a group of patients. I am responsible for setting patient care goals and then directing my team to achieve the goals. I make those patient care goals the focus of my team's efforts. Patient care is rendered with the assistance of subordinates, including Certified Nurse Assistants (CNAs), nursing student externs, and occasional high school student volunteers. Communication is the key to a successful team. A recent patient typifies how I interact with my team.

An elderly nonverbal patient with a history of schizophrenia was admitted to our surgical unit for dehydration. She was in need of total care especially with respect to hygiene, which had been neglected. She was dependent on staff to turn and position her. Her level of awareness suggested she was unable to use a call light for help.

This patient challenged staff for a variety of reasons. First, due to multiple other health problems, she was not a candidate for surgery. This placed her among the patients who don't really "fit" the surgical unit where she was admitted. Nonetheless, my goal was to advocate for comfort care with her physician while also encouraging subordinates to provide quality care even though the goal was not cure with this particular patient. The patient's inability to communicate verbally added to the challenge. It was unclear how aware the patient was of the care she was receiving. Her nonverbal status blocked her ability to dialogue. This caused us to rely on nonverbal cues. Respect for patients with or without their verbal feedback is essential. The CNA and I tackled the bed bath together. Teamwork kept the focus on the goal for the patient, which was to optimize comfort and maintain skin integrity. It allowed me to complete a thorough assessment and to model desired communication with the patient whom I addressed by name. I inquired whether she was in pain, to which she responded with twisting motions. I continued the one-way conversation, attempting to clarify what her nonverbal responses meant. She pointed to her shoulder, so we repositioned her and she settled down, resting quietly. As is often the case, the CNA willingly returned to reposition the patient with confidence the remainder of the shift. The patient's inability to verbalize needs was perceived as less of a barrier once we were successful overcoming it together.

I find that CNAs will often volunteer to complete entire tasks they feel capable of performing independently. They also have the confidence that they will not be expected to handle clinical situations for which they do not feel qualified. This mutual respect for each other is essential to an ongoing working relationship. They honor the standard of care and will often complete tasks, going above and beyond what I ask. For example, later in the afternoon, the CNA returned to the patient and washed and braided her hair.

*(continues)*

**Real World Interview** (*continued*)

Since this same patient would not likely use the call light, I also explained our goal to the high school student volunteer and I asked her to check the patient's position whenever she went by the room. I instructed her to let me know if the patient appeared uncomfortable, assuring her that I would reposition the patient as needed. The student expressed that she thought it was cool how nurses communicate with patients who can't talk. I believe through effective communication our team achieved the goal of optimizing this patient's comfort in spite of many potential barriers.

*Lari Summa,* RN, BSN

**Attending.** **Attending** involves active listening. Active listening requires that the nurse pay close attention to what the patient is communicating, both verbally and nonverbally. The nurse pays close attention during communication, looking for congruence between what is said and how it is said. Attending involves the nurse's nonverbal cues. Facing the person and maintaining eye contact are two skills that facilitate attending. If possible, sitting down and leaning forward sends a message that the nurse is willing to listen. Distracting behaviors, such as tapping one's foot, send a message that the nurse is not interested in the message. Therefore, these types of behaviors should be avoided.

**Responding.** **Responding** entails verbal and nonverbal acknowledgment of the sender's message. When the nurse nods affirmatively while listening, the nurse is responding nonverbally that the message has worth. A response can be as simple as an acknowledgment that the message was received, e.g., "I hear you." Sometimes, however, responding involves more. Two verbal skills that elevate the level of responding are questioning and restating. Questioning allows the nurse to clarify the message by asking related questions. Restating involves restating what the nurse believes to be the important points. These techniques refine perceptions and enhance understanding.

**Clarifying.** **Clarifying** helps the communication become clear through the use of such techniques as restating and questioning. For example, if the nurse does not understand a patient's account of a presenting complaint, the nurse can respond with, "I lost you there." Perhaps the nurse tries to process information that is confusing or conflicting. The nurse can restate what was heard in an effort to clarify the information. Questioning and restating are used not only to respond, but also to clarify.

**Confronting.**   **Confronting** means to work jointly with others to resolve a problem or conflict. Given that definition, it is a very effective means of resolving conflict. See the discussion of conflict later in this chapter. Confronting involves, first of all, identifying the conflict, which can arise from perceived or real differences. A nurse might identify a conflict with a simple, "We have a problem here." Next, the problem is clearly delineated so that those involved understand what it is and what it is not. Then using knowledge and reason, attempts are made to resolve the problem. The goal is to achieve a win-win solution where both party's needs are met. This sounds easier to do than it sometimes is because emotions can get in the way and cloud reason. Cooling off periods are sometimes needed between problem identification and conflict resolution. Acceptable motives for confronting are to resolve conflict, to further growth, and to improve relationships (Ruthman, 2003). See Table 3-2 for additional communication skills.

## STOP AND THINK

You are having a coffee break with another nurse who mentions a problem she is having with care delivery. The nurse is not sure how to solve it. You want to be helpful and supportive and yet avoid giving advice. Ask the nurse if she can describe the problem fully for you. Do not interrupt. Then, ask the nurse some questions about the problem and seek clarification until you are clear on the problem and the nurse has fully described it. Do not give advice. Use your communication skills, such as attending, clarifying, and responding, and ask the nurse such things as, tell me more about that; what did you think about it, and so forth, until you are both clear on the issue. At the end of this process, you can just finish by relaxing for the rest of your break or you can ask the nurse, "Do you want advice about your problem?"

Many times, this process will help the nurse with the problem solve it himself or herself. If she does want advice, you can give her some suggestions if you are comfortable doing so. Do you think this process can strengthen people's ability to find answers to their problems? Do you think this process would be helpful to you in working with others on the unit? Do you think this process would be helpful to you in solving any other problems? Do you think this approach honors people's integrity and ability to solve their own problems?

Adapted from M. Parsons (personal communication, 2003). San Antonio, TX.

**TABLE 3-2**
*ADDITIONAL COMMUNICATION SKILLS*

| | |
|---|---|
| Supporting | Siding with another person or backing up another person, e.g., "I can see how you would feel that way." |
| Focusing | Centering on the main point, e.g., "So your main concern is . . ." |
| Open-ended questioning | Allows for person-directed responses, e.g., "How did that make you feel?" |
| Providing information | Supplies one with knowledge one did not previously have, e.g., "It's common for people with pneumonia to be tired." |
| Listening and using silence | Allows for observation of the communication process |
| Reassuring | Restores confidence or removes fear, e.g., "I can assure you that tomorrow . . ." |
| Expressing appreciation | Shows gratitude, e.g., "Thank you," and "You are so thoughtful." |
| Using humor | Provides relief and gains perspective; may also cause harm, so use carefully. |
| Conveying acceptance | Makes known that one is capable or worthy, e.g., "It's okay to be concerned about that." |
| Asking related questions | Expands listener's understanding, e.g., "How painful was that experience for you?" |
| Broad openings | Initiates conversation, e.g., "What has been going on with you?" |
| Restating | Provides feedback and lets the patient know that the nurse understood the message, e.g., "Are you saying that you are angry?" |
| Reflection | Presents themes that have emerged through a series of interactions, e.g., "So, you are feeling depressed because no one called you yesterday?" |
| Informing | Provides facts or recommendations, e.g., "The medications must be taken at 0900 daily." |
| Suggesting | Presents new ideas, e.g., "Have you considered asking for a day off?" |

Adapted from Ruthman, 2003. Communication in Kelly-Heidenthal, PL, Nursing Leadership and Management, Delmar, 2003, Clifton Park, NY.

# CULTURE AND DELEGATION

Our culture grows increasingly diverse. This diversity reduces the likelihood that patients, nurses, and other health care staff will share a common cultural background. In turn, the number of safe assumptions about beliefs and practices decreases and the probability for misunderstanding increases. For example, shortly after delivering a baby, women are often hungry and thirsty. Some cultures believe that in order for women to restore their energies appropriately, women are to eat hot foods and beverages while others believe cold foods and beverages are appropriate. A well-intentioned nurse who does not consult the patient about her preferences may arrange culturally inappropriate nourishment. Culture encompasses different groups' beliefs and practices by gender, race, age, economic status, health, and disability (Ruthman, 2003). Giger and Davidhizar, 1999, outline six phenomena that must be considered when delegating to staff with culturally diverse backgrounds. These phenomena are communication, space, social organization, time, environmental control, and biological variations.

## Communication

Communication, the first cultural phenomena, is greatly affected by cultural diversity in the work force. Elements of communication, such as dialect, volume, use of touch, context of speech, and kinesics (such as gestures, stance, and eye behavior) all influence how messages are sent and received (Giger and Davidhizar, 1999). For example, if a nurse is talking to a UAP in a loud voice, it can be interpreted as anger. However, the nurse may be from a cultural background that always speaks loudly. The nurse may not be angry at all. Alternately, a nurse, because of cultural upbringing, may speak in a quiet, nondirective way that could be wrongly perceived as lacking authority.

## Space

Cultural background influences the space that individuals maintain between themselves and others. Some cultures prefer physical closeness when speaking while other cultures prefer more distance to be maintained between people. Ineffective delegation can take place when an individual's space is violated. Some stand too close when speaking. Conversely, some members of a group may feel left out if they are not sitting close to the delegator. They may not feel included or important.

## Social Organization

In different cultures, the social support in a person's life varies from support from one's own family, friends, and environment, to support from collegial relationships within the work place. If a staff member looks to other staff at work for social support, those staff will have difficulty fulfilling any tasks delegated to them that could threaten their social organization.

## Time

Another cultural phenomenon affecting delegation is the concept of time. Have you heard people say, "They are on their own time schedule?" Some people tend to react and move more slowly whereas other people move quickly and are prompt in meeting deadlines.

Giger and Davidhizar (1999) describe different cultural groups as being past, present, or future oriented. Past-oriented cultures focus on their tradition and its maintenance. For example, these cultures invest much time into preparation of food that is traditional even though the food can be bought prepared in a store. Present-oriented cultures focus on day-to-day activity. For example, a present-oriented culture works hard for today's wages but does not plan for the future. Future-oriented cultures worry about what might happen in the future and prepare diligently for a potential problem, perhaps financial or health related. A nurse delegator should always communicate not only duties to be completed but also their deadline, so all personnel can be clear about performing their duties in a timely fashion.

## Environmental Control

Giger and Davidhizar (1999) define environmental control as people's perception of control over their environment. Some cultures place a heavy weight on fate, luck, or chance, believing, for example, that a patient is cured from cancer based on chance. They may think the health care treatment had something to do with the cure, but was not the sole cause of the cure. They may stress the role of fate as an external locus of control.

How staff perceives their control of the environment may affect how they delegate and perform duties. Staff with an internal locus of control is geared toward setting goals, taking more control, having self-initiative, and not requiring assistance in decision-making. They believe in taking action and not relying on fate.

Staff with an external locus of control may wait for others and luck or fate to determine their actions and tell them what to do. The nurse delegator working with this group will spell out carefully what the staff must complete.

## Biological Variations

The sixth cultural phenomenon is biological variations. Biological variations are the biological differences between racial and ethnic groups. These biolog-

## STOP AND THINK

*The Luck Factor,* published in 2003, authored by R. Wiseman, discusses research that illustrates luck as something that can be learned if one pays attention to four principles:

- Lucky people create, notice, and act on the chance opportunities in their life.
- Lucky people make successful decisions by using their intuition and gut feeling.
- Lucky people's expectations about the future help them fulfill their dreams and ambitions.
- Lucky people are able to transform their bad luck into good fortune.

Do you agree with Wiseman's findings? Can you use your "luck" to improve your nursing career? Your life? Discuss.

ical variations include physiological differences, physical stamina, and susceptibility to disease. For example, delegating the nursing care of a comatose patient who is greater than 300 pounds and who requires frequent turning to a small nurse who can't physically handle the patient should be considered when delegating. Perhaps this patient should be assigned to two nurses. Likewise a pregnant nurse would not be assigned to a patient with radium implants because of the risks radium may have to the baby and mother. Biological variations are considered for the sake of both the health care providers and the patient.

# THE PROFESSIONAL ROLE OF THE NURSE

Nurses have a legal and professional responsibility to deliver quality nursing care to their patients. Experts in the social sciences are considered the authorities on what makes an occupation a profession. Although there is some variation in actual criteria of a profession, there is general agreement in several areas:

- Professional status is achieved when an occupation involves a unique practice that carries individual responsibility and is based upon theoretical knowledge.
- The privilege to practice is granted only after the individual has completed a standardized program of highly specialized education and has demonstrated an ability to meet the standards for practice.

- The body of specialized knowledge is continually developed and evaluated through research.
- The members are self-organizing and they collectively assume the responsibility of establishing standards for education in practice. They continually evaluate the quality of services provided in order to protect the individual members and the public.

There is a trend in recent years to call every occupation a profession. Have you heard of professional computer operators, professional automobile mechanics, professional teachers, professional nurses, and professional lawyers? There has been a tendency to confuse professionalism and profession. The term "professionalism" generally refers to an individual's commitment and dedication to the occupation. Professionalism often also refers to the attitude, appearance, and conduct of the individual. Whether an occupation is a profession requires more analysis. Figure 3-2 refers to some charac-

| Flexner, 1915 | Bixler and Bixler, 1959 |
|---|---|
| • Intellectual activities<br>• Activities based on knowledge<br>• Activities can be learned<br>• Activities must be practical<br>• Techniques are teachable<br>• A strong organization exists<br>• Altruism motivates the work | • Specialized body of knowledge<br>• Growing body of knowledge<br>• New knowledge used to improve education and practice<br>• Education takes place in higher education institutions<br>• Autonomous practice<br>• Service above personal gain<br>• Compensation through freedom of action, continuing professional growth, and economic security |
| **Pavalko, 1971** | **Public Law 93-360 on Collective Bargaining** |
| • Work based on systematic body of theory and abstract knowledge<br>• Work has social value<br>• Length of education required for specialization<br>• Service to public<br>• Autonomy<br>• Commitment to profession<br>• Group identity and subculture<br>• Existence of a code of ethics | • Predominantly intellectual work<br>• Varied work requirements<br>• Requires discretion and judgment<br>• Results cannot be standardized over time<br>• Requires advanced instruction and study |

**Figure 3-2** Characteristics of a Profession (Courtesy, Mitchell, GM, and Grippando, PR, Nursing Perspectives and Issues, Delmar, Albany, NY, 1994)

---

**Professional Values:**

| | | |
|---|---|---|
| Caring | Freedom | Justice |
| Altruism | Esthetics | Truth |
| Equality | Human dignity | Ethical |
| Nonjudgmental | | |

**Professional Behaviors and Attributes:**

| | |
|---|---|
| Appearance | Stress management |
| Time-management skills | Self-evaluation |
| Self-discipline | Initiative |
| Maintenance of licensure/certification | Motivation |
| Participation in institutional/community | Creativity |
|   activities | Effective communication |
| Participation in continuing education | |
| Political awareness | |
| Reading professional journals | |
| Participation in nursing research | |

---

**Figure 3-3** Possible Characteristics of a Professional (Courtesy, Mitchell, GM, and Grippando, PR, Nursing Perspectives and Issues, Delmar, Albany, NY, 1994)

teristics of a profession identified by different sources. Figure 3-3 lists some of the values, behaviors, and attributes that may be exhibited by a "professional" (Mitchell and Grippando, 1993).

# STOP AND THINK

As a beginning nurse, you are interested in research that identifies the benefits to consumers of quality nursing care. These benefits include less incidence of "failure to rescue" patients. Benefits also include lower rates of nurse-sensitive patient outcomes, such as the death of a patient with life-threatening complications, like pneumonia, shock, cardiac arrest, urinary tract infection, gastrointestinal bleeding, sepsis, or deep vein thrombosis (Needleman, Buerhaus, Mattke, Stewart, and Zelevinsky, 2002).

Ask yourself, how does your nursing practice identify essential dimensions of nursing? See Box on following page. How do you define nursing? How do you identify your distinctive nursing services? Benefits to consumers? Cost of your services? Have you ever witnessed a "failure to rescue" or witnessed a nurse "rescuing" a patient? Would the patient have lived if the nurse was not present? Is nursing a profession? Use Table 3-3 to develop your own professional style.

## FOUR ESSENTIAL DIMENSIONS OF NURSING

1. *Nursing* is "attention to the full range of human experiences and responses to health and illness without restriction to a problem-focused orientation" (American Nurses Association, 1995, p. 6).

2. *Distinctive services nurses provide* include, but are not limited to, coordinating total patient care, completing ongoing health assessment, and advocating for quality care for patients. Nursing is perhaps the only profession whose focus is the patient's total health care.

3. *Benefits to consumers* include lower rates of nurse sensitive outcomes (defined in research study as death of a patient with one of the following life-threatening complications: pneumonia, shock, cardiac arrest, urinary tract infection, gastrointestinal bleeding, sepsis, or deep vein thrombosis, and "failure to rescue") (Needleman, Buerhaus, Mattke, Stewart, and Zelevinsky, 2002).

4. *Costs of nursing services* vary according to the care setting and role of the nurse. Primary care delivered by nurse practitioners and services provided by certified nurse mid-wives cost less than the same care delivered by physicians (Shi & Singh, 2001, pp. 138–139).

## TABLE 3-3
## DEVELOPING A PROFESSIONAL STYLE

1. Assess your current education and experience.
2. As you start your new nursing role, review the following on your unit:
   - Ten most common medical diagnoses
   - Ten most common nursing diagnoses
   - Ten most common medications and IV solutions
   - Ten most common diagnostic tests
   - Ten most common laboratory tests
   - Ten most common nursing and medical interventions and treatments
3. Set goals for any additional education and experience that you may need.
4. Review your own job description and the role and the job description of nursing and other healthcare and medical staff you work with.
5. Identify the names and contact information of all nursing, medical, and health care staff that you work with.
6. Discuss delegation with your preceptor and observe how the preceptor delegates to others.
7. Observe the impact of delegation on both the delegate and the person delegated to.

*(continues)*

**Table 3-3** (*continued*)

8. Remember the golden rule; do unto others as you would want them to do unto you.
9. Recognize that, under the law, the RN holds the responsibility and accountability for nursing care.
10. Practice assertiveness and work at being direct, open, and honest in your new role.
11. Exercise your power with kindness to all.
12. Hold others accountable for their responsibilities as spelled out in their job description.
13. Be open to performance improvement feedback about your personal delegation style.
14. Modify your communication approach to fit the needs of patients, staff, and yourself.

# POTENTIAL BARRIERS TO COMMUNICATION

The nurse who can identify potential barriers to communication will be better equipped to avoid them or to compensate for them. Some of the most common barriers in addition to culture are gender, anger, incongruent responses, conflict, and thought distortions.

## Gender

Gender interferes with communication when men and women lack understanding that they may process information differently. In general, some men are more interested in using communication to solve problems and get a task done. Some women talk to make a point, give and receive emotional support, relieve tension, or discover a point. Every person has a natural blend of male and feminine characteristics (Gray, 2001).

Gender differences and patterns do not preclude working together. Rather, they require that both sides realize that others may have different preferences and make accommodations so that effective communication and working relationships result.

Gender differences have been attributed, in part, to gender socialization where males may have been provided with more opportunities to develop confidence and assertiveness than females. The feminist movement and increased sexual equality in western society, in general, have lessened traditional sociological patterns of competitiveness and decisiveness in men and passivity and nurturing in women. However, remnants of the traditional model persist, particularly in health care settings. Nurses who lack assertiveness and confidence are encouraged to acquire the requisite skills to be assertive and confident in order to be an effective patient advocate and also to communicate in a confident manner (Ruthman, 2003).

## Anger

**Anger** is a universal, strong feeling of displeasure that is often precipitated by a situation that frustrates or prevents a person from attaining a goal. Anger is influenced by one's beliefs. Ellis (2002) describes anger as an irrational response that arises from one of four irrational ideas: (1) thinking that the treatment one received was awful (awfulizing), (2) feeling that one can't stand having been treated so irresponsibly and unfairly (can't-stand-it-itis), (3) believing that one should not, must not behave as he did (shoulding and musting), and (4) thinking that because one acted in a terrible manner, he is a terrible person (undeservingness and damnation). Ellis maintains that beliefs remain rational as long as the evaluation of the action does not involve an evaluation of the person. Rational and appropriate responses are feelings of disappointment. Anger, on the other hand, can be unmanageable and self-defeating. Ellis believes that we all have the ability to choose our response to anger.

### FOUR IRRATIONAL IDEAS WHICH LEAD TO ANGER

Awfulizing

Can't-stand-it-itis

Shoulding and musting

Undeservingness and damnation

Ellis, 2002.

Anger can be dealt with in one of several ways. Three methods that may work from time to time but have serious and potentially destructive drawbacks are: denying and repressing anger, which may lead to resentment; expressing anger, which may lead to defensiveness on the part of the respondent; and turning the other cheek, which may lead to continued mistreatment and lack of trust. Since anger stems from carrying things further and viewing the situation as awful, terrible or horrible, Ellis (2002) advocates disputing irrational beliefs. Anger can stem from deep-seated feelings of unassertiveness. Assertion involves taking a stand while aggression involves putting another person down. If unassertiveness is the source of anger, then a solution is to learn to act assertively.

## STOP AND THINK

Nurses who practice assertiveness are direct, honest, and appropriate. They say, "I need you to do . . ." rather than, "You should do. . . ." The next time you work in the clinical area, note how nurses interact with their staff, other nurses, physicians, and practitioners. Do the nurses always speak assertively? Is it always easy to do? Is being assertive part of being a professional nurse? Is it possible to meet your patient's needs if you are not assertive?

## Incongruent Responses

When words and actions in a communication don't match the inner experience of self and/or are inappropriate to the context, the response is incongruent. Some common incongruent responses are blaming, placating, being super reasonable, and using irrelevant information for decision-making.

**Blaming** is finding fault or error and occurs when a response lacks respect for others' feelings. For example, a nurse who attributes a medication error to an overloaded assignment might blame the nurse who made the assignment, accusing that "It's all her fault." This can be avoided by speaking up when the assignment is made and standing up for one's rights while respecting the rights of others.

Placating is soothing by concession and occurs when one lacks self-respect. For example, a nurse who consents to a patient assignment that she believes is unfair or unsafe just to keep the peace is placating. Placating can be overcome by paying attention to one's own needs and by negotiating what one believes to be a fair and safe assignment.

Being super reasonable is to go beyond reason and demonstrate lack of respect for others' and one's own feelings. The nurse above, who when approached by the house supervisor, agrees to whatever solution is offered has become super reasonable when she says, "You're always right, I'll do whatever you need." This ineffective approach can be sidestepped by clarifying goals and yet considering each other's feelings when arriving at a solution.

Finally, using irrelevant information for decision-making shows lack of respect for others' and one's own feelings. A nurse who challenges a colleague's abilities based solely on their out of work activities or political preference is using irrelevant information. Likewise, arguing against a colleague's ability to function as a charge nurse because of an incident that occurred a year prior during the nurse's orientation may be irrelevant. Respecting feelings and the context within which an event occurred can avert irrelevance (Ruthman, 2003).

## Conflict

Conflict arises when ideas or beliefs are opposed. Not surprisingly, it occurs at different levels, such as the interpersonal and organizational level. Conflict resolution is another way to resolve conflict besides the confronting method discussed earlier in this chapter. In conflict resolution, the nature of the differences and the reasons for the differences are considered. Differences arise for an array of reasons. Variations in facts, goals, and methods to achieve the goals, values, or standards, as well as priorities all contribute to these differences (Kinney & Hurst, 1979). Conflict resolution typically occurs using different approaches. See Table 3-4.

## Thought Distortions

Research on thinking processes has shown that people sometimes make mistakes in the way they perceive information and think about the world around them. For example, when people are somewhat depressed, their automatic thoughts are loaded with distorted thinking. If one can recognize these thought distortions, one can begin to turn life in a more positive direction. See Table 3-5.

## STOP AND THINK

Sometimes you may work with staff that is difficult. These staff can include staff who usually work in another setting; staff who are more knowledgable than you; staff who are older than you; staff who think they are better than they are; and staff who are defensive when you ask them to do something. With all these staff, it can help to develop strategies that identify your performance expectations clearly and involve them in the work that needs to be done. This is useful with all types of staff, those that are easy to work with and those that are difficult. How can you work to improve your ability to communicate your performance expectations clearly to staff that you work with?

**TABLE 3-4**

*SUMMARY OF CONFLICT RESOLUTION TECHNIQUES*

| Conflict Resolution Technique | Advantages | Disadvantages |
|---|---|---|
| Accommodating— smoothing or cooperating. One side gives in to the other side | One side is more concerned with an issue than the other side; stakes not high enough for one group and that side is willing to give in | One side holds more power and can force the other side to give in; the importance of the stakes are not as apparent to one side as the other; can lead to parties feeling "used" if they are always pressured to give in |
| Avoiding—ignoring the conflict | Does not make a big deal out of nothing; conflict may be minor in comparison to other priorities; allows tempers to cool | Conflict can become bigger than anticipated; source of conflict might be more important to one person or group than others |
| Collaborating—both sides work together to develop optimal outcomes | Best solution for the conflict and encompasses all important goals to each side | Takes a lot of time; requires commitment to success |
| Competing—forcing; the two or three sides are forced to compete for the goal | Produces a winner; good when time is short and stakes are high | Produces a loser; may leave anger and resentment on losing side |
| Compromising— each side gives up something and gains something | No one should win or lose but both should gain something; good for disagreements between individuals | May cause a return to the conflict if what is given up becomes more important than the original goal |

*(continues)*

**Table 3-4** (*continued*)

| Conflict Resolution Technique | Advantages | Disadvantages |
|---|---|---|
| Confronting— immediate and obvious movement to stop conflict at the very start | Does not allow conflict to take root; very powerful | May leave impression that conflict is not tolerated; may make something big out of nothing |
| Negotiating—high-level discussion that seeks agreement but not necessarily consensus | Stakes are very high and solution is rather permanent; often involves powerful groups | Agreements are permanent, even though each side has gains and losses |

## TABLE 3-5
### *THOUGHT DISTORTIONS*

| Thought Distortion | Example |
|---|---|
| All-or-nothing thinking: seeing things only in absolutes | If I leave this job, no one will respect me. |
| Overgeneralization: interpreting every small setback as a never-ending pattern of defeat | Everyone here is so smart; I'm a real loser. |
| Dwelling on negatives: ignoring multiple positive experiences | I made a mistake. I'm not good enough to be a nurse. |
| Jumping to conclusions: assuming that others are reacting negatively without definite evidence | I don't know why I study. Everyone thinks I'm going to fail NCLEX anyway. |
| Pessimism: automatically predicting that things will turn out badly | It's only a matter of time before everything falls apart for me. |
| Reasoning from feeling: thinking that if one feels bad, one must be bad. | My head hurts because I'm a bad person. I deserve it! |
| Obligations: living life around a succession of too many "shoulds," "shouldn'ts," "musts," "oughts," and "have tos." | I should marry Mike. Everyone likes him. |

Compiled with information from Frisch, NC, & Frisch, LE, Psychiatric Mental Health Nursing. Delmar, Clifton Park, NY 1998.

## Additional Barriers to Communication

Other barriers to communication are seen in Table 3-6.

# OVERCOMING COMMUNICATION BARRIERS

DuBrin (2000) has identified nine strategies and tactics for overcoming communication barriers. See Table 3-7.

In addition to these strategies, it is helpful to use stress management techniques to avoid the anxiety associated with communication barriers. See Table 3-8.

# HELPFUL AND NON-HELPFUL ROLES IN COMMUNICATION

In any group, there are bound to be both participants who are helpful and those who are not helpful in their behaviors. Sometimes these behaviors are

**TABLE 3-6**
*BARRIERS TO COMMUNICATION*

| | |
|---|---|
| Offering False Reassurance | Promising something that can't be delivered. |
| Being Defensive | Acting as though one has been attacked. |
| Stereotyping | Unfairly categorizing someone based on his or her traits. |
| Interrupting | Speaking before the other person has completed their message. |
| Stress | A state of tension that gets in the way of reasoning. |
| Inattention | Not paying attention. |
| Unclear Expectations | Asking for ill-defined tasks or duties that makes successful completion unlikely. |
| Denial | Denying the reality of threatening situations. |

Adapted from Ruthman, 2003, Communication, in Kelly-Heidenthal, PL, Nursing Leadership and Management, Delmar, 2003, Clifton Park, NY.

**TABLE 3-7**

*OVERCOMING COMMUNICATION BARRIERS*

| | |
|---|---|
| Understand the receiver | • Ask yourself, what's in it for the other person<br>• Work to develop understanding of the other person's needs |
| Communicate assertively | • Be direct<br>• Explain ideas clearly and with feeling<br>• Repeat important messages<br>• Use various communication channels, e.g., written, e-mail, verbal, and so on |
| Use two-way communication | • Ask questions<br>• Communicate face to face |
| Unite with a common vocabulary | • Define the meaning of important terms, such as high quality, so that everyone understands their meaning |
| Elicit verbal and nonverbal feedback | • Request and offer verbal feedback often<br>• Document important agreements<br>• Observe nonverbal feedback |
| Enhance listening skills | • Pay attention to what is said, what is not said, and to the nonverbal signals<br>• Continue listening carefully even when you don't like the message<br>• Give summary reflections to assure understanding, for example, "You say you are late giving medication because the pharmacy did not deliver meds on time."<br>• Engage in concluding discussions, such as, "Has your unit been late with medications due to problems with pharmacy deliveries before?"<br>• Ask questions to explore problems<br>• Paraphrase a speaker's words to decrease miscommunication rather than blurting out questions as soon as the other person finishes speaking |
| Be sensitive to cultural differences | • Know that cultural communication barriers exist<br>• Show respect for all workers<br>• Minimize use of jargon specific to your culture<br>• Be sensitive to cultural etiquette, such as, use of first names, eye contact, hand gestures, personal appearance |

*(continues)*

**Table 3-7** (*continued*)

| | |
|---|---|
| Be sensitive to gender differences | • Be aware that men and women may have some differences in communication style, for instance, men may call attention to their accomplishments and women may tend to be more conciliatory when facing differences<br>• Know that male-female stereotypes often don't fit the person you are working with<br>• Avoid barriers by knowing that differences exist and don't take things personally<br>• Males can improve communication by showing more empathy and females by becoming more direct |
| Engage in meta-communication | • Communicate about your communication to resolve a problem, such as, "I'm trying to get through to you, but either you don't react to me or you get angry. What can I do to improve our communication?" |

Adapted from DuBrin, AJ, The Active Manager, South-Western Pub., United Kingdom, 2000.

unconsciously acted out. At other times, a group member is quite clear and focused about the role that they are playing, such as the aggressor. In any case, it is imperative that the astute nurse leader be aware of everyone's roles and use excellent communication skills to facilitate the team's work. See Table 3-9.

## Destructive or Difficult Behaviors

Nurses who delegate may occasionally work with people who are not interested in good communication and accomplishing a task. Strategies for coping with these difficult people are identified in Table 3-10.

Other destructive behaviors that people may exhibit on a health care team include being the disapprover or blocker of others' suggestions; being a recognition seeker; being a self-confessor of personal, nongroup-oriented feelings or comments; being a playboy or playgirl; being a dominator or help seeker; or using the group to meet personal needs or to plead special interests (Northouse & Northouse, 1992). These destructive behaviors can interfere with the health care team meeting the patient's needs.

## TABLE 3-8
### STRESS MANAGEMENT TECHNIQUES

| | | |
|---|---|---|
| Meditate | Do relaxation exercises | Be polite to all |
| Think peaceful thoughts | Do something different for lunch | Take a walk |
| See things as others might | Give yourself a pat on the back | Read |
| Forgive your mistakes | Join a support group | Join a club |
| Do not procrastinate | Talk about your worries | Sing a song |
| Set realistic goals | Be affectionate | Forgive and forget |
| Do a good deed | View problems as a challenge | Listen to music |
| Vary your routine | Get or give a massage | Take a hot bath |
| Appreciate what you have | Say a prayer | Call an old friend |
| Focus on the positive | Expect to be successful | Laugh more |
| Let go of the need to be perfect | | |

Adapted from Koren, M. E., Healthy Living: Integrating Personal and Professional Needs, in Kelly-Heidenthal, P. (2003), Nursing Leadership and Management. Clifton Park, NY, Delmar.

## TABLE 3-9
### COMMON MEMBER ROLES

Common member roles in groups fit into three categories: group task roles, group maintenance roles, and self-oriented-roles.
- *Group task roles* help a group develop and accomplish its goals. Among these roles are the following:
  - Initiator-contributor: Proposes goals, suggests ways of approaching tasks, and recommends procedures for approaching a problem or task
  - Information seeker: Asks for information, viewpoints, and suggestions about the problem or task
  - Information giver: Offers information, viewpoints, and suggestions about the problem or task
  - Coordinator: Clarifies and synthesizes various ideas in an effort to tie together the work of the members
  - Orienter: Summarizes, points to departures from goals, and raises questions about discussion direction
  - Energizer: Stimulates the group to higher levels of work and better quality

*(continues)*

**Table 3-9** (*continued*)

- *Group maintenance roles* do not directly address a task itself but, instead, help foster group unity, positive interpersonal relations among group members, and development of the ability of members to work effectively together. Group maintenance roles include the following:
    - Encourager: Expresses warmth and friendliness toward group members, encourages them, and acknowledges their contributions
    - Harmonizer: Mediates disagreements between other members and attempts to help reconcile differences
    - Gatekeeper: Tries to keep lines of communication open and promotes the participation of all members
    - Standard setter: Suggests standards for ways in which the group will operate and checks whether members are satisfied with the functioning of the group
    - Group observer: Watches the internal operations of the group and provides feedback about how participants are doing and how they might be able to function better
    - Follower: Goes along with the group and is friendly but relatively passive
- *Self-oriented roles* are related to the personal needs of group members and often negatively influence the effectiveness of a group. These roles include the following:
    - Aggressor: Deflates the contributions of others by attacking their ideas, ridiculing their feelings, and displaying excessive competitiveness
    - Blocker: Tends to be negative, stubborn, and resistive of new ideas, sometimes in order to force the group to readdress a viewpoint that it has already dealt with
    - Recognition seeker: Seeks attention, boasts about accomplishments and capabilities, and works to prevent being placed in an inferior position in the group
    - Dominator: Tries to assert control and manipulates the group or certain group members through such methods as flattering, giving orders, or interrupting others

Adapted from Bartol K, and Martin, D, 1998, 3rd Ed., Management, McGraw-Hill, Boston, MA.

**TABLE 3-10**
*STRATEGIES FOR COPING WITH DIFFICULT PEOPLE*

| Personality Type | Coping Strategies |
|---|---|
| Criticizer | Don't argue—it will add only fuel to the fire! Ask for input and practice active listening by reflecting on what you heard. Give criticizers a project to which they can directly contribute. |
| Passive person | Engage in communication, ask direct questions, and ask for direct responses. |
| Detailer | Allow the detailer to give details at certain points in a group. Begin with the objective for the group, repeat information when necessary, summarize. |
| Controller | Keep focused on the task at hand; note any inconsistencies in the controller's conversation. |
| Pleaser | Let pleasers know that their comments are safe from attack, and that their opinions are valued. |

Adapted from Polifko-Harris, K, 2003, in Kelly-Heidenthal, PL, Nursing Leadership and Management, Delmar, 2003, Clifton Park, NY.

## STOP AND THINK

Sometimes, in your role as a nurse on the unit, you must counsel people who are not doing their job. It helps if you have told them your expectations clearly, such as, your goals, directions, and the needed outcomes. If their performance is still lacking, you may need to talk with them further. Try to identify any areas of genuine strength that needs to be continued and enhanced. Then identify areas needing improvement. Do you think this technique would begin to solve the issue? Have you ever worked with someone who was not doing his or her part of a task? How did you resolve it? Did the situation improve? What would you do differently next time?

# MYERS-BRIGGS PERSONALITY TYPES

If a team is to succeed, it is helpful to get the right blend of personalities, experience, and temperaments to work toward a common goal. An astute nursing team leader will keep in mind that some personality types complement others. A tool that some organizations use to assist them in devising effective work teams and team building is the Myers-Briggs Type Indicator (MBTI), a psychological testing instrument that identifies different personality types. Major personality types according to the MBTI fall into four pairs of categories and indicate how people:

1. Focus their attention: are they an Introvert (I) or an Extrovert (E)?
2. Take in information from their surroundings: are they Sensing (S) or Intuitive (N)?
3. Prefer to make decisions: are they Thinking (T) or Feeling (F)?
4. Relate to the external world: do they have Judging (J) characteristics or Perceiving (P) characteristics?

The MBTI categorizes individuals into each one of these four pairs of categories, for example, a person may be an Extrovert, Sensing, Feeling, Judging Type (ESFJ), or any one of sixteen different possible combinations of the four category pairs. See Table 3-11.

A critical point to make in using the MBTI is that in the MBTI, there is no right or wrong personality type. Everyone is different and these differences should be respected (Keirsey & Bates, 1978). The MBTI should only be used for guidance, not for placing people into distinct categories. If fact, most people are not at one end of the continuum or the other. Most are somewhere on a scale. For example, a person may be 60% Extrovert and 40% Introvert, 20% Sensing and 80% Intuitive, 90% Thinking and 10% Feeling, and 30% Judging and 70% Perceiving. The MBTI just provides one additional piece of information about people. Its results are not "locked in stone." See Figure 3-4.

## STOP AND THINK

Go to one of the web sites in the "Exploring the Web" section. Take the MBTI. What did you discover about yourself? Were you surprised with the results? Ask your coworkers to take the MBTI. Ask them to tell you what type they think you are. If they are willing, ask them to tell you what type they believe they are. Does their interpretation of themselves agree with how you would identify them? What did you learn about yourself from their interpretation of you? What did you learn about your coworkers? Remember in interpreting the results, there is no one "best type." Each type has its strengths and opportunities for improvement.

## WORKPLACE COMMUNICATION

How individuals communicate depends, in part, on where communication occurs and in what relationship. Patterns of communication in the workplace

## TABLE 3-11
## *MYERS-BRIGGS TYPE INDICATOR CATEGORIES*

| | |
|---|---|
| Introverts | Private, energized by working alone and may be anxious in group settings. They think before acting. Prefer 1:1 relationships. |
| Extroverts | Get energized around a crowd and do their best work when there is a lot of excitement requiring multi-tasking. They act before thinking. |
| Sensors | Take in information through their five senses and rely on this input to make practical, realistic decisions. They trust the facts and focus on details. Memory recall of the past is highly detailed. |
| Intuitives | Idealistic. They trust their hunches and focus on the big picture. Memory recall emphasizes patterns, contexts, and connections. Comfortable with ambiguous, fuzzy data. |
| Thinkers | Logical, objective, and analytical when making decisions. They are fair and employ cause and effect reasoning. They accept conflict as a natural, normal part of working with people. |
| Feelers | Are able to place themselves in a situation and look at how they or someone else may view an outcome before making a decision. Feelers are concerned with keeping harmony in the environment. They are unsettled by conflict and seek consensus. |
| Judgers | Prefer to live in an organized, scheduled world, making and keeping a plan and lists. They want to know just the essentials and take action quickly. Judgers naturally use deadlines and goals to manage their life. |
| Perceivers | Being spontaneous, casual, and flexible are the hallmarks of this personality. They feel confined when made to keep to a schedule. They postpone decisions and find it hard to meet deadlines that interfere with their freedom and flexibility. |

Compiled from *Gifts Differing* by I. Briggs Myers and P. B. Myers, 1995, Palo Alto, CA: Davies-Black.

are sensitive to organizational factors that define relationships. Nurses have diverse roles and relationships in the workplace that call for different communication patterns with superiors, co-workers, and other nursing and medical practitioners.

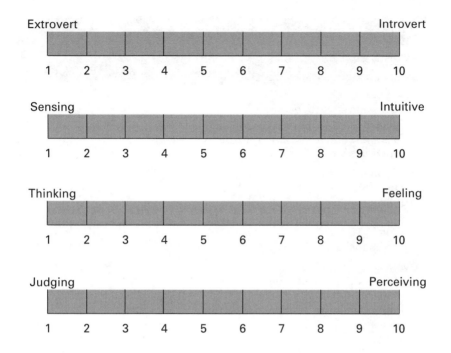

**Figure 3-4** Myers-Briggs Type Indicator Scale

# Communicating with Superiors

Communicating with a superior about problems can be intimidating, especially for a new nurse. Observing professional courtesies is an important first step. For instance, if there is time, begin by requesting an appointment to discuss a problem. This demonstrates respect for the superior and allows for the conversation to occur at an appropriate time and place. If a problem is more pressing, report it to your supervisor as soon as possible. This report usually starts with the charge nurse who may in turn need to communicate the problem to his or her supervisor. Don't hesitate to communicate up the organizational chain of command discussed in Chapter 1 if you feel the problem remains unresolved. It is usually best to start with your direct supervisor. Be prepared to state the concern clearly and accurately. Provide supporting evidence. State a willingness to cooperate in finding a solution and then match behaviors to words. Persist in the pursuit of a solution (Ruthman, 2003). See Table 3-12 for a checklist for working with your boss. You may find it helpful to use a personal process recording to examine and improve your communications. See Table 3-13.

**TABLE 3-12**
*HOW TO IMPROVE YOUR ABILITY TO WORK WITH
YOUR BOSS*

Know your boss's
- Goals and Objectives
- Pressures
- Strengths and weaknesses and blind spots
- Working style

Understand your own
- Objectives
- Pressures
- Strengths and weaknesses
- Working style
- Predisposition toward dependence on authority figures

Develop a relationship that
- Meets both your objectives and styles
- Keeps your boss informed
- Is based on dependability and honesty
- Selectively uses your boss's time and resources

Adapted from Gabarro, JJ, and Kotter, JP, Managing your boss, Harvard Business Review, May–June, 1993, 150–157.

# Communicating with Co-Workers

Nurses work directly or indirectly with a wide variety of people. One of the challenges in working in health care is the interdisciplinary focus that revolves around patient care delivery. Sovie (1992) discusses the need for high quality teams in health care that have a specific purpose, and that contribute to the organization's overall outcomes performance. A registered nurse is directly responsible for the care of the patient, but that care includes ensuring that the correct medical and nursing orders are carried out, such as did the correct medication dosage get transcribed, did the UAP document the intake and output accurately for the shift, did the LPN complete the ordered treatments, was the discharge planning coordinated with the social worker and case manager, did the pharmacist distribute the medications, does the family understand how to dress the patient's wound, and finally, does the patient understand the discharge instructions? Nurses depend on their co-workers in many ways to collectively provide quality patient care. Nowhere is this more important than in the acute care setting where nursing services are nonstop around the clock.

## TABLE 3-13
### *PROCESS RECORDING EXCERPT*

| Interaction | | Communication Technique Used | Evaluation |
|---|---|---|---|
| Nurse preceptor: | What has been going on with you this week? | Broad Opening | Permits nurse to begin with what is important at the moment |
| Nurse 2: | I have been thinking a lot about my job. I feel like I don't delegate care the way that I should. | | |
| Nurse preceptor: | You are not delegating care well enough? | Restating | Provides chance for nurse 2 to expand on thoughts. |
| Nurse 2: | No. I think that I should be doing better. | | |
| Nurse preceptor: | So, you think you should be doing better? | Reflection | Returns nurse 2 to feelings. Nurse 2 is then able to talk about past experiences. |
| Nurse 2: | Yes, I find it hard to tell someone else what to do. I worry that my patients won't get good care if I don't learn delegation as I can't do all the nursing care myself. I need the help of others. | | |
| Nurse preceptor: | Others? | Clarification | Allows nurse manager to seek information, yet encourages nurse 2 to go on. |
| Nurse 2: | Yes, I need some more help to get better at delegation. | | |
| Nurse preceptor: | OK, let's work together. | | |

An excellent guide for directing communication with co-workers is the golden rule, "do unto others as you would have them do unto you." As a nurse who will be responsible for overseeing others' work, a valuable perspective for you to maintain is that all members of the team are important to successfully realize quality patient care. Communication between nurses and co-workers will usually involve delegating. Offering positive feedback such as, "I appreciate the way you interacted with Mr. T. to get him to ambulate twice this shift" goes a long way towards team building, and it improves co-workers' sense of worth. Nurses also have an opportunity to act as teachers to co-workers. Often in a hospital setting nurses teach by example. Demonstrating the desired behavior allows the co-worker to copy the behavior. It is important to allow time for return demonstrations to evaluate that the co-workers have learned the intended skill. For example, as the nurse, you may demonstrate how to position a patient with special needs, encouraging the co-worker to assist and ask questions. The next time repositioning is indicated, accompany the co-worker and observe his or her ability to successfully complete the task. Offer constructive feedback. Be patient. Remember your own learning curves when mastering new skills and behaviors and allow those you supervise the opportunity to grow. Be open to the possibility that co-workers, particularly those with experience, may have a few pearls of wisdom to share with you as well (Ruthman, 2003).

## BUILDING A SUCCESSFUL TEAM

Davis, Hellervik, Sheard, Skube, and Gebelein (1996) offer the following suggestions for building a successful team:
- Value the contributions of all team members: all members are critical to the success of the team regardless of their position on the team.
- Encourage interaction among group members: know when verbal and nonverbal behavior is appropriate and inappropriate and keep the flow of communication going.
- Discourage "we versus they" thinking: build teamwork that encourages inter-team participation and relationships.
- Involve others in shaping plans and decisions: involving the total team in the problem solving and decision making will strengthen any suggested changes made by the team because the entire team is able to support the decisions.
- Acknowledge and celebrate team accomplishments: publicly and frequently acknowledge positive contributions by team members, and keep the team members abreast of the positive changes they are actively involved in making.
- Evaluate your effectiveness as a team member: being an effective team leader includes being an effective team member. Are you carrying your weight, or are you expecting others to carry out your directives?

## REAL WORLD INTERVIEW

I work as a nurse technician at a local hospital. As a technician, we are allowed to perform procedures that we have learned in nursing education clinical experiences under the supervision of a RN. One day I walked up to the nurse's station and a nurse handed me the supplies to start an IV. She said the patient in room 5432 needed an IV started and that it would be a good experience for me. I responded that I had never started an IV before and that I was not allowed to do so. The nurse said "Don't worry; I will walk you through it." I said, I'm sorry, but I do not feel comfortable. The nurse rolled her eyes at me and walked away as she was talking rudely under her breath.

*Rachel Golonka, Nurse Technician*

### SELECTED TIPS ON CIVILITY

- Smile.
- Give praise.
- Admit you are wrong.
- Let others be kind to you.
- Keep your voice low in public places.
- Do not ridicule, humiliate, or demean others.
- Show consideration.

## STOP AND THINK

Nurses need to be aware that different staff in the workforce may see things differently based on their age differences. For example, young staff people, called Millennials or Nexters, often do exactly what is asked and work primarily to earn money to spend. Slightly older staff, called Generation X, save, save, save, and work to eliminate the task. Baby boomers like to buy now, pay later, and work very efficiently. Veterans or matures are older staff who work fast, sacrifice, and are very thrifty (Zemke, Raines, & Filipczak, 2000). These staff may have a hard time working together toward a goal. Do you see any of these age differences affecting the clinical area where you work? How can nurses bridge these differences?

## Communicating with other Nursing and Medical Practitioners

Communicating with other practitioners and physicians need not be intimidating or stressful. The nurse's goal is to strive for collaboration, keeping the patient goal central to the discussion. Collaboration allows both parties to be satisfied. It involves seeking creative, integrative solutions while also working through emotions. Cardillo (2001) gives several tips on working with doctors. She suggests that it is useful to establish rapport and introduce yourself to the doctors that you work with. Don't be intimidated. You and the doctor are both on the health care team to meet the patient's goals. At least one study has indicated that when nurses and doctors work together, patient's death rates or readmission rates decrease (Baggs & Ryan, 1990). Both you and the doctor are important to your patient's welfare.

## LITERATURE APPLICATION

**Citation:** Greene, J. (2002). The medical workplace. No abuse zone. *Hospitals and Health Networks, 76*(3), 26, 28.

**Discussion:** An astounding number of health care workers, 62% to 96%, say they experienced or witnessed abusive behavior in the past year from a supervisor, a doctor, or even a patient. For example, a nurse working the night shift gets a medication order she can't read and calls the physician at 2 A.M. for clarification. He yells at her and hangs up without answering the question. The nurse is afraid to call back and gives a fatal dose of the wrong drug.

This article discusses guidelines for a five-stage process to rid health care workplaces of abusive behavior. Deborah Anderson, President of Respond 2 Inc., St. Paul, Minnesota, is developing the guidelines in conjunction with the Hennepin Medical Society, Minneapolis, Minnesota. The Respond 2, Inc. 5-Stage Process includes: building a team that meets monthly, surveying employees with an assessment tool about their experiences with workplace abuse, devising a plan to deal with workplace abuse, evaluating outcomes with a resurvey, and infusing the workplace with an atmosphere of collegiality by changing policies and procedures that affect culture, hiring, employee orientation, training, reporting processes, performance evaluation, and appropriate patient safety and quality related initiatives. In developing this five-stage process, it is imperative that strong support be in place from the leaders of the organization.

**Implications for Practice:** This 5-stage Process can be very useful in developing a No Abuse Workplace.

Show respect and consideration for the doctors you work with but don't be a doormat. Give due respect and expect the same from them. Present information in a straightforward manner, clearly delineating the problem, supported by pertinent evidence. This is especially important when reporting changes in patient conditions. See Table 3-14 for a tool to organize patient information prior to calling another practitioner or doctor for assistance. Nurses are responsible for knowing classic symptoms of conditions, orally apprising the practitioner or physician of changes, and recording all observations in the chart (Sanchez-Sweatman, 1996).

Cardillo (2001) suggests that nurses be assertive. Don't call a doctor and say, "I'm sorry to bother you." You are not bothering her. It is her job to answer and you are doing your job by calling her. If you don't understand something, ask questions. Many doctors love to teach. Be honest and up front. Tell the doctor if something is new to you.

| TABLE 3-14 *TOOL TO ORGANIZE INFORMATION FOR CALLING ANOTHER PRACTITIONER OR PHYSICIAN FOR ASSISTANCE* | |
| --- | --- |
| Room Number and Name: | |
| All Diagnoses: | |
| Allergies: | |
| Current Medications and IV fluids: | |
| Current and baseline vitals, status of airway, breathing, and circulation, level of consciousness, urine output, pain level: | |
| Current Problem: | |
| Potential outcome of problem for patient: | |
| Action needed from practitioner that you are calling: | |
| Urgency of call: | |
| Time of call and response of practitioner: | |
| Office or exchange called/messages left: | |

## REAL WORLD INTERVIEW

A second shift occupational health nurse working in a factory setting was presented with a patient who entered the nursing office complaining that he didn't feel good. The nurse's initial assessment, including vital signs, revealed that the only abnormality was an elevated blood pressure. In this situation, as in any clinical situation, it is important to distinguish the urgent from the nonurgent. With hypertensive patients, it is important to realize that an urgent situation is suggested by evidence of acute end organ damage. Specifically, in this situation, it was important to know whether the patient was experiencing altered sensorium, headache, visual disturbance, chest pain, or dyspnea. The presence of any of these findings should be communicated to the physician and would dictate urgent transport to the hospital. In their absence, the patient can be referred for more elective blood pressure control.

In any clinical situation, such as the one above, the nurse can facilitate communications by being organized and objective. Be prepared to cover the basics such as the patient's chief complaint, his vital signs, his medications, and any changes from baseline. Know why you are worried about observed changes and communicate this to the MD.

*John C. Ruthman,* MD

When you call the doctor, if they do not respond appropriately or are out of line, you might say, "I don't appreciate being spoken to in that way," or "I would appreciate being spoken to in a civil tone of voice and I promise to do the same with you," or something similar. Calfee (1998) offers suggestions for handling telephone miscommunications. For example, if a physician hangs up, document that the call was terminated, fill out an incident report, and notify your supervisors. If the physician gives an inappropriate answer or gives no orders, for example, for a patient complaint of pain, document the call, the information relayed, and the fact that no orders were given. In addition, document any other steps that were taken to resolve the problem. If the practitioner does give you a verbal or telephone order, be sure to repeat the order back to the practitioner and document after the written order, Telephone Order Repeated Back (TORB) or Verbal Order Repeated Back (VORB).

Cardillo suggests that nurses seek clarification from the doctor if an order is unclear. If an order is inappropriate or incorrect, rather then saying, "This order does not seem appropriate for this patient," which would likely put the doctor on the defensive, try "Teach me something, Dr. Jones, I've never seen a dose of Lopressor that high. Can you explain the therapeutic dynamics to me?" or "Dr. Smith, I can't for the life of me figure out why you ordered a brain scan on this patient. Can you help me out here?" This approach usually results in the doctor either reevaluating an order or changing it. If the doctor doesn't change an order that you think is inappropriate or you can't reach the doctor, let your supervisor know and follow the chain of command guidelines of the agency where you work (LaBarre, 2003).

> In all cases, nurses must remember that since the RN owes a duty directly to the patient, blindly relying on another nursing or medical practitioner's judgment is not permissible for the RN.

# LITERATURE APPLICATION

**Citation:** Johnson, L. (2004). Shortage of nurses putting patients at risk: Unions push for limits on patient loads in hospitals. *Associated Press.* Retrieved March 29, 2004 from http://msnbc.msn.com

**Discussion:** Across the country, nurses unions are pushing hospitals and lawmakers for limits on patient loads. And hospitals are trying to recruit and keep more nurses, all with good reason. Too few nurses can cost patients their health and sometimes their lives, study after study shows.

A shortage of nurses is a factor in about one-fourth of patient injuries or deaths in hospitals, according to the Joint Commission on Accreditation of Healthcare Organizations' 2002 report.

The prestigious Institute of Medicine says long work hours and fatigue contribute to errors. Its November 2003 report recommends a ban on nurses working longer than 12 hours a day.

A 2002 study by Harvard and Vanderbilt university researchers, examining millions of 1997 hospital cases, found preventable deaths and patient complication rates were up to nine times higher in hospitals where the most care was given by licensed practical nurses and aides, not better-trained RNs.

For each additional patient over four assigned to a nurse, the risk of dying after surgery rose 7 percent, according to a 2002 survey of 168 Pennsylvania hospitals by Linda Aiken, director of the Center for Health Outcomes and Policy Research at the University of Pennsylvania School of Nursing.

Finding enough qualified RNs will remain tough: The U.S. Department of Health and Human Services projects the current shortage of a few hundred thousand RNs could hit 750,000 by 2020, as aging Baby Boomers need more care and the nursing workforce gets older.

*(continues)*

**Literature Application** (*continued*)

But in Washington and states from New Jersey to Oregon, nurses' unions are ramping up battles for new laws or contracts setting minimum nurse-patient ratios. Local unions have been fighting for—and increasingly winning—contracts that limit patient loads or that put nurses on committees that set staffing guidelines.

Many nursing groups are looking to California as a model for nurse ratios. In January, it enacted the nation's first hard-and-fast ratios, ward by ward. An RN may care for six patients at most, and only four in the ER and two in critical care units.

Six other states—Florida, Kentucky, Nevada, Oregon, Texas and Virginia—have enacted staffing regulations but not ratios, and 18 states introduced some staffing legislation last year, according to the American Nurses Association.

**Implications for Practice:** Nurses who are interested in quality nursing practice will be interested in the solutions to the nursing shortage being proposed.

# REVIEW QUESTIONS

1. The nurse delegated to an experienced UAP to reposition a particular patient. After two hours had gone by, the nurse asked the UAP if the patient had been turned. The UAP replied, "No, I'm sorry, but I have not gotten to it yet." What should the nurse have done to ensure this task was completed in a timely fashion when the nurse first delegated the task to the UAP?
   A. Explained the procedure to the UAP.
   B. Assisted the UAP in the procedure.
   C. Realized this procedure is outside the UAP's scope of practice.
   D. Informed the UAP of the time frame within which the procedure was to be completed.

2. The RN delegated to an experienced LPN to pass medications to patients in rooms 2035–2040. Several hours later, one of the patients complained to the RN that they had not received their medications. What should the nurse do at this time?
   A. Disregard the patient's complaint.
   B. Follow the LPN during the medication process.
   C. Ask all the patients if they have received their medications.
   D. Explore the patient's complaint with the LPN to determine what happened.

3. An RN asks the UAP to take a set of vital signs on a patient who has just had an arterial venous shunt placement. The RN reminds the UAP not to take the blood pressure (BP) on the operative side. An hour later the RN finds the deflated blood pressure cuff on the operative arm of the patient. The UAP has done this before and has been counseled about it. What should the RN do first?
   A. Assess the patient's condition.
   B. Avoid asking this UAP to take BPs in the future.
   C. Discuss the situation with the UAP and the supervisor.
   D. Find the UAP and review the importance of taking the blood pressure on the non-operative side.

4. A new graduate RN received an unfamiliar treatment order from the MD. How should the nurse proceed?
   A. Refuse to do the treatment.
   B. Do the treatment to the best of the nurse's ability.
   C. Inform the MD and then proceed to do the treatment.
   D. Inform the MD and ask the MD or charge nurse for assistance in doing the procedure.

5. What part of the communication process returns input to the sender?
   A. Feedback
   B. Message
   C. Receiver
   D. Sender

6. Which of the following characteristics pertains to verbal communication?
   A. Eye contact
   B. Nodding
   C. Smiling
   D. Tone of Voice

7. Which of the following skills involves active listening and is a very important skill used by nurses to gain an understanding of the patient's message?
   A. Attending
   B. Clarifying
   C. Confronting
   D. Responding

8. Why must nurses be concerned about barriers to communication?
   A. Because they enhance interactions
   B. So that they can use them when communicating
   C. Nurses don't need to be concerned
   D. So that they can overcome them

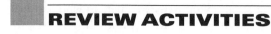

# REVIEW ACTIVITIES

1. The charge nurse apologizes as she informs you that your assignment includes the "problem UAP" on the unit. What communication skills will you use to enhance communication with this UAP? How will you avoid barriers of communication with this UAP?

2. You found out that you passed your NCLEX-RN last month. When you report for your evening shift, you discover you are assigned to be the team leader. What communication skills will you use to communicate with the other nursing and medical health care staff?

3. Check out this site for the MBTI. Decide what MBTI type you are and ask a friend or colleague to identify what type they think you are. It is always informative to discover if you see yourself the way that others see you.

   http://www.personalitypathways.com/type_inventory.html

4. Mary is feeling more comfortable with the knowledge level she needs to safely care for her patients. She would like to improve her ability to work with and delegate to the UAP that she works with. How can she proceed? How can Mary use the 4 C's of Communication discussed in Table 3-1 to delegate effectively?

5. Colleen, an RN, has been working on the unit for almost a year now and is working as a preceptor to Josie, a new graduate nurse. Colleen remembers what it was like to be a novice and is trying to help Josie adapt to her new role. Colleen recalls that it took her a long time to do anything when she started and she tells Josie this fact.

   Colleen also notes that her skills increased as she assumed more personal responsibility for learning new skills and as she became comfortable with both the policies and procedures of the unit and the job descriptions of herself and her staff. Colleen tells Josie to expect it to take a while to be skilled in her role. Colleen suggests that Josie use Table 3-3 to guide her in her role preparation. How can you use Table 3-3 to take personal responsibility for developing your professional nursing role?

# EXPLORING THE WEB

1. More information about the MBTI tool can be found at
   http://www.typelogic.com (Accessed 10-02) or
   (http://www.keirsey.com/search for sixteen roles) (Accessed 10-02)
   or (http://www.humanmetrics.com)
   (http://www.personalitypathways.com)

2. Check these web sites
   For online journal articles
   http://www.medscape.com/search for online nursing journals

   Nursing articles are available online at
   www.nursingcenter.com
   and
   http://www.nursingmanagement.com

   Check this site.
   http://www.nsna.org/

   Check this guide to education and careers in nursing which includes the most comprehensive directory of nursing schools with full school profiles, and detailed nursing questions and answers.
   www.allnursingschools.com

   Check out this University of Michigan site for time management tips. (http://www.umich.edu/search for stress manager)

## REFERENCES

Baggs, J. G., & Ryan, S. A. (1990). ICU nurse-physician collaboration and nursing satisfaction. *Nursing Economics, 8*(6), 386–392.

Bartol, K., & Martin, D. (1998). *Management* (3rd ed.). Boston, MA: McGraw-Hill.

Calfee, B. E. (1998). Making calls to the physician. *Nursing, 10,* p. 17.

Cardillo, D. W. (2001). *Your first year as a nurse.* Roseville, CA: Prima.

Ellis, A. (2002). *Anger: how to live with and without it.* New York, NY: Kensington Publishing Corporation.

Frisch, N. C., & Frisch, L. E. (1998). *Psychiatric mental health nursing.* Albany, NY: Delmar.

Giger, J. N., & Davidhizer, R. E. (1999). *Transcultural nursing.* Baltimore, MD: Mosby.

Gray, J. (2001). *Mars and Venus in the workplace: A practical guide for improving communication & getting results at work.* New York: Harper Collins.

Keirsey, D., & Bates, M. (1978). *Please understand me: Character and temperament types.* Del Mar, CA: Prometheus Nemesis Books.

Kinney, M., & Hurst, J. (1979). *Group process in education.* Lexington, MA: Ginn Customs.

Koren, M. E. (2003). *Healthy living: Integrating personal and professional needs.* In P. Kelly-Heidenthal, *Nursing leadership and management.* Clifton Park, NY: Delmar.

LaBarre, L. (2003). *Your first job.* In P. Kelly-Heidenthal. *Nursing leadership and management.* Clifton Park, NY: Delmar.

Lasswell, H. D. (1948). *The structure and function of communication in society.* In L. Bryson (Ed.), *The communication of ideas.* Lanham, MD: Rowman and Littlefield, Institute for Religious and Social Studies.

Needleman, J., Buerhaus, P., Mattke, S., Stewart, M., & Zelevinsky, K. (2002). Nurse-staffing levels and the quality of care in hospitals. *New England Journal of Medicine, 346*(22), 1715–1722.

No Abuse Zone. Hospitals and Health Networks. March, 2002. 26, 28.

Northouse, P. G., & Northouse, L. L. (1992). Health Communication: Strategies for Health Professionals (2nd ed.). Norwalk, CT: Appleton and Lange.

Ruthman, J. (2003). *Personal and interdisciplinary communication.* In P. Kelly-Heidenthal. *Nursing leadership and management.* Clifton Park, New York: Delmar.

Sanchez-Sweatman, L. (1996). Communicating with physicians. *Canadian Nurse 92*(8): 49–50.

Sovie, M. (1992). Care and service teams: A new imperative. *Nursing Economic$, 10*(2), 94–100.

White, L., & Duncan, G. (2002). *Medical-surgical nursing* (2nd ed.). Clifton Park, NY: Delmar.

Yoder-Wise, P. S. (2002). *Leading and managing in nursing* (3rd ed.). St Louis, MO: Mosby.

Zemke, R., Raines, C., & Filipczak, B. (2000). *Generations at work: Managing the clash of veterans, boomers, Xers, and nexters in your workplace.* New York, NY: Pearson Custom Publishing.

Zerwekh, J., & Claborn, J. (2002). *Nursing today: Transition and trends.* St. Louis, MO: Saunders.

## SUGGESTED READINGS

Baker, C., Beglinger, J., King, S., Salyards, M., and Thompson, A. (2000). Transforming negative work cultures. *JONA, 30*(7/8), 357–363.

Bradley, J. C., & Edinberg, M. A. (1986). *Communication in the nursing context.* Norwalk, CT: Appleton-Century-Crofts.

Chant, S., Jenkinson, T., Randle, J., & Russell, G. (2002). Communication skills: Some problems in nursing education and practice. *Journal of Clinical Nursing, 11*(1), 12–21.

Davidhizar, R., & Giger, J. N. (2001). Teaching culture within the nursing curriculum using the Giger-Davidhizar Model of Transcultural Nursing Assessment. *Journal of Nursing Education, 40*(6), 282–284.

Dowd, S. B., Giger, J. N., & Davidhizar, R. (1998). Use of Giger and Davidhizar's Transcultural Assessment Model by health professions. *International Nursing Review, 45*(4), 119–122, 128.

Giger, J. N., & Davidhizar, R. (2002). The Giger and Davidhizar Transcultural Assessment Model. *Journal of Transcultural Nursing, 13*(3), 185–188.

Teytelman, Y. (2002). Effective nursing documentation and communication. *Semin Oncol Nurs., 18*(2), 121–127.

Walczak, M. B., & Absolon, P. L. (2001). Essentials for effective communication in oncology nursing: assertiveness, conflict management, delegation, and motivation. *Journal of Nurses Staff Development, 17*(2), 67–70. Corrected and republished in: *Journal of Nurses Staff Development, 2001, 17*(3), 159–162.

Williams, C. A., & Gossett, M. T. (2001). Nursing communication: Advocacy for the patient or physician? *Clin Nurs Res. 10*(3), 332–340.

# CHAPTER 4

Autonomy means decision control over the kind and degree of service a client will receive. It involves a conscious decision about what will and what will not be done when there is more work than available time. Control over time use is a key aspect of professional nurse practice (Roxane Spitzer-Lehmann, 1996).

# Time Management and Setting Priorities

## OBJECTIVES

*Upon completion of this chapter, the reader should be able to:*

1. Discuss general time management techniques.

2. Analyze the use of professional nursing and personal time.

3. Review time wasters.

4. Discuss behaviors of perfectionists vs. pursuers of excellence.

5. Discuss effective use of available time.

6. Describe setting priorities for safe patient care.

7. Discuss shift report and how to make assignments.

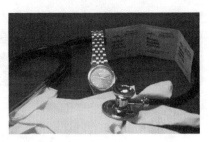

*Colleen has just completed her medical-surgi-cal orientation as a new graduate registered nurse. This evening is her first solo shift. But she is not really alone. Colleen and Mary, the other Registered Nurse (RN), and two unlicensed assistive personnel (UAP), are responsible for 12 patients in this section of the unit. Currently there are 11 patients in this section of the unit and a new admission is on the way. The patient from the recovery room has just returned from thyroid surgery, the dinner trays are arriving, and Colleen has medications to pass. Just as the dinner trays arrive, the daughter of Mrs. Glusak, Room 2509, runs out to Colleen and states that her mom seems more confused and is incontinent. Her mother has just pulled out her own IV and it is leaking on the floor.*

*What would you do first if you were Colleen?*

*How can Colleen manage her time and set priorities?*

(See patient description, p. xxii)

M any people become nurses out of idealism. They want to help others by meeting their needs. Unfortunately most new graduates find it impossible to meet all, or even most, of their patients' needs. Needs tend to be unlimited while time is limited. In addition to direct patient care responsibilities, there are shift responsibilities, charting, doctor's orders to be transcribed or checked, medications to be given, and patient reports to be given.

New graduates often go home feeling totally inadequate. They wake up remembering what they did not accomplish. One young nurse, with tears in her eyes, shared that once, when she answered a call bell late in her shift, the patient requested a pain medication. She went to the narcotics cabinet to get the medication, but was interrupted by an emergency situation. When she arrived home, she was so exhausted that she fell asleep rapidly, only to awaken with the realization that she had not returned with her patient's medication. Her guilt was tremendous. She had gone into nursing to relieve pain, not to ignore it.

Using time management and setting priorities allows the new nurse to prioritize care, decide on outcomes, and perform or delegate the most important interventions first. Time management skill is not just important for nurses on the job. It is important for their personal lives as well. Time management allows nurses to make time for fun, friends, exercise, and professional development (Maloney, 2003). This chapter discusses general time management tips, the setting of priorities, the importance of setting goals, and illustrates one way to analyze professional and personal time. It discusses behaviors of perfectionists versus pursuers of excellence and discusses shift report, patient rounds, and how to make assignments.

## GENERAL TIME MANAGEMENT TECHNIQUES

**Time management** has been defined as "a set of related common-sense skills that helps you use your time in the most effective and productive way possible" (Mind tools, 1995–1998). In other words, time management allows us to achieve more with the available time we have. Time management requires self-examination of what pursuits are really important, analysis of how time is currently being used, and assessment of the distractions that have been siphoning time from more important pursuits.

Time management requires a shift from being busy to getting things done, a shift from focusing on the process of work to focusing on achieving a good work outcome. A busy frenzy is often reinforced with sympathy and assistance from others. Too often this frenzied behavior is accomplishing very little, because it is not directed at the right outcome. There is a simple principle, the **Pareto principle**, which states that 20% of focused effort results in 80% of desired outcomes or results, or conversely that 80% of unfocused effort results in 20% of results. See Figure 4-1.

The Total Quality Management (TQM) movement invoked Pareto's Principle, formulated by Vilfredo Pareto in the late 1800s, as a strategy for balancing life and work (Fryxell, 1997; Graham, 1998; Koch, 1999). Effective time management requires that a shift is made from unfocused activities that require 80% of time for achieving 20% of desired results to one of planned and

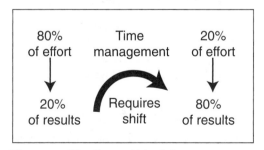

**Figure 4-1** The Pareto Principle

focused activities that use only 20% of time or input to achieve 80% of desired outcomes (Maloney, 2003).

## STOP AND THINK

When you ask overworked nurses why they did not plan their shift, they often say that they did not have time. Do you think they really did not have time? Jumping into your work without a plan is like starting a journey without looking at a map. How much time would you waste if you just started driving? Think about this the next time you work. What outcomes do you want to achieve? What is your plan for achieving these outcomes?

If time management is so easy, why do so many people continue at a crazy, hurried pace? There are several possible explanations for this. Perhaps they do not know time management skills, they think that they do not have time to plan, they do not want to stop to plan, or perhaps they love crisis (Mind tools, 1995–1998).

## Outcome or Goal Orientation

The first step in any time management and priority setting strategy is to shift from focusing on the process of work and being task oriented to focusing on achieving outcomes or goals. Goals or outcomes must be determined. It is best to break these outcomes down into achievable smaller outcomes that are steps toward the larger outcomes. Often, large goals and outcomes cannot be achieved immediately. The goals should be written down and should remain flexible. There may come a time when a desired outcome may no longer be realistic or should be shifted to a more realistic outcome as circumstances change (Reed & Pettigrew, 1999).

## ANALYSIS OF NURSING TIME

Analysis of nursing time use is important in developing a plan to effectively use time. Nurses cannot possibly know how to better plan their time without knowing how they currently use time. When keeping track of time, it is important to consider the value of a nurse's time as well as the use of the time.

## Value of Nursing Time

Nurses often undervalue their time. Consider salary and benefits. Benefits are frequently forgotten, but they comprise 15% to 30% of total cost per employee. If a nurse is making $18.00 an hour, benefits add $2.70 to $5.40 to the hourly cost of a nurse's time. The value of nursing time in this example, excluding what the organization is paying in workman's compensation and payroll taxes, is $20.70 to $23.40 per hour. The organization has also invested in nurse recruitment, orientation, and development besides these costs.

Nursing time is a valuable commodity. Keeping this in mind will be invaluable when considering work that can be delegated to personnel who receive less compensation or when considering spending time on completing a task that does not support achieving an outcome (Maloney, 2003).

## Use of Time

Numerous studies have shown how nurses use their time. Most studies have been done on acute care nurses, since they comprise a majority of nurses. Only 30% to 35% of nursing time is spent on direct patient care (Scharf, 1997). Twenty-five percent of a nurse's time is spent on charting and reporting, and the remaining time is spent on admission and discharge procedures, professional communication, personal time, and providing care that can be provided by unlicensed personnel such as transportation and housekeeping (Upenieks, 1998). Urden and Roode (1997) summarized various work sampling studies to show that RNs spend 28% to 33% of their time on direct patient care, defined as activities performed in the presence of the patient and/or family. They spend 42% to 45% of time on indirect care activities which includes all activities done for an individual patient, but not in the patient's presence. They spend 15% on unit-related activities, which include all unit general maintenance activities; and 13% to 20% on personal activities, which include activities that are not related to patient care or unit maintenance. See Figure 4-2.

Given such a distribution of nurse's time, a shift in the use of time could have a major impact on outcomes. If non-nursing personnel instead of nurses could perform non-nursing activities, about 48 minutes per nurse per shift could be re-directed toward essential nursing responsibilities (Prescott, Phillips, Ryan, & Thompson, 1991).

How do you use your time? Memory and self-reporting of time have been found to be unreliable. Nurses are often unaware of the time spent working, socializing with colleagues, making and drinking coffee, snacking and so on. Self-reporting of time is not recommended for estimating the total number of activities or the average time an activity takes to complete (Burke, McKee, Wilson, Donahue, Batenhorst, & Pathak, 2000).

## Activity Log

An **activity log** is a time management tool that can assist the nurse in determining how both personal and professional time is used. The activity log (Table 4-1) should be used for several days.

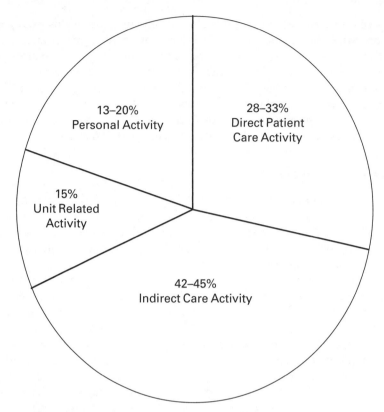

**Figure 4-2** Use of RN Time (Adapted from Urden, L, and Roode, J, 1997, Work Sampling, JONA, 1997)

Behavior should not be modified while keeping the activity log. The nurse should record every activity, from the beginning of the day until the end. Review of this log will illuminate time use as well as time wasted. Analysis of the log will allow the separation of essential activities from activities that can be delegated to someone else (Grohar-Murray & DiCroce, 1997; Sullivan & Decker, 2001).

After completing the activity log, a nurse needs to consider all activities that have been completed, how much time each activity took, what outcome was achieved by performing the activities, and whether the activities could have been delegated to another. Notice your most energetic time of day. Activities that take focus and creativity should be scheduled at high-energy times and dull, repetitive tasks at low energy times.

Use the activity log to examine relationships between eating patterns, rest patterns, and energy levels. If a person is tired and non-productive after a large lunch, she or he should break the lunch down into several smaller snacks.

## TABLE 4-1
### ACTIVITY LOG

| Time | Name of Activity | Outcome Desired | Delegate To Another? |
|------|------------------|-----------------|----------------------|
| 0500 | Treadmill | Fitness | No |
| 0530 | Shower and breakfast | Cleanliness and Nutrition | No |
| 0600 | Drive to work | Arrive at work | No |
| 0630 | | | |
| 0700 | Report and patient rounds | Identify and assess patients | No |
| 0730 | Give report to UAP | Safe patient care | No |
| 0800 | Patient breakfast | Patient nutrition | Yes |
| 0830 | Baths and bed making | Patient bathing and providing clean beds | Assign to UAP |
| 0900 | Pass medications | Safe medication delivery | No |
| 0930 | Dressing change | Prevent infection | Assign to LPN |
| 1000 | | | |
| 1030 | | | |
| 1100 | | | |
| 1130 | | | |
| 1200 | | | |
| 1230 | | | |
| 1300 | | | |
| 1330 | | | |
| 1400 | | | |
| 1430 | | | |
| 1500 | | | |
| 1530 | | | |
| 1600 | | | |
| 1630 | | | |
| 1700 | | | |
| 1730 | | | |
| 1800 | | | |
| 1830 | | | |
| 1900 | | | |
| 1930 | | | |
| 2000 | | | |
| 2030 | | | |
| 2100 | | | |

Scheduling time for proper rest, exercise, and nutrition allows for quality time. When considering these questions, ask yoursolf, how would the Pareto principle apply? Has 20% of the effort resulted in 80% of outcome achievement? If the activities have not achieved the desired outcomes, the nurse needs to re-prioritize. Do this analysis with both your professional and personal time.

## Create More Time

There are several ways to create time. You can prioritize, perform a task yourself, delegate work to others, or hire someone else to do it. Other ways are to avoid time wasters, eliminate chores or tasks that add no value, or to get up earlier in the day. See Table 4-2 for time wasters that apply to your personal and professional time.

Avoiding these time wasters will help you achieve excellence. You want to achieve excellence, not perfection! See Table 4-3.

When a person delegates a task they cannot completely control when and how the task is completed. Initially, it may take more time to delegate to others to do a chore than to do it oneself, but this investment of time should save time and energy in the future. If a chore is boring and mundane, it makes more sense to work an hour more at a job one enjoys in order to pay for someone else to do work you find unrewarding or boring.

Getting up one hour earlier in the day can free up 365 hours, or approximately nine additional weeks a year. This extra time can be used to enrich life. After several days of rising an hour earlier, an individual may feel tired and respond to the fatigue by going to bed a little earlier (Mind tools, n.d.-a). This may be a good strategy for many people, especially those who are not productive in the evening and spend time doing activities that are minimally rewarding such as watching television. If a person does not try to get to bed earlier, though, and the end result of getting up early is fatigue, the strategy is not beneficial (Maloney, 2003).

## LITERATURE APPLICATION

**Citation:** Estrich, S. (1997). *Making the case for yourself*. New York, NY: Riverhead Books.

**Discussion:** Author discusses the importance of taking care of oneself and following a plan to eat properly and exercise regularly. She highlights the need to live one's life in a healthy manner. She suggests putting the same effort into planning your health as you do into planning your other professional endeavors.

*(continues)*

## Literature Application (*continued*)

**Implications for Practice:** This text highlights the importance of taking responsibility for living a healthy life and making a plan to achieve it. Nurses who take good care of themselves have the strength to take good care of their patients.

## TABLE 4-2
### *TIME WASTERS*

Are you a time waster? We all sometimes behave in ways that sabotage the best of plans. Following are some examples of time wasters along with some strategies to help you reclaim those wasted hours.

1. Clutter: Wisdom holds that you can save one hour each day just by clearing your work area of clutter and keeping it clean. Organize your work area and take a few minutes at the end of your shift to prepare it for the next shift.
2. Interruptions: Intrusions into your work time (from either people or things) can be real time wasters. Try the following:
   - Learn to say, "No." You do not have to agree to every request. Learn to pick your involvements carefully and pick those that are most important to reaching your goals.
   - Put your answering machine on at home and turn the telephone's ringer off. Identify a time to listen and respond to messages.
   - Open your mail over the garbage can. Respond, delegate, or throw it out.
   - Organize your papers. Keep your notebooks, calendar, and telephone lists in one three ring binder so you have your essentials together.
3. Procrastination: This refers to intentionally putting off or delaying something that should be done. Procrastination is a time waster because it does not afford effective use of time. Time management is not necessarily finishing everything at one sitting, but rather, scheduling time to return to the task until you complete it; whereas procrastination is intentionally delaying the task without good cause or a plan to complete it in a time-efficient manner. Breaking the task down into manageable segments and rewards will encourage you to return to it again and again until it is complete.
4. Perfectionism: Very often we do not stick to a plan because it does not give us immediate results or the results we expected. Perfectionism affects your time-management plan by prohibiting you from accepting anything less than perfection; it also damages your positive attitude by setting unrealistic expectations of yourself. Focus on your positive accomplishments, look for ways to improve, accept your failures, and build on your experiences.

Courtesy, White, L, Critical Thinking in Practical/Vocational Nursing, 2000, Delmar.

**TABLE 4-3**

***BEHAVIORS OF PERFECTIONISTS VS. PURSUERS OF EXCELLENCE***

| Perfectionists | Pursuers of Excellence |
|---|---|
| • Hate criticism | • Learn from failure |
| • Are devastated by failure | • Welcome criticism |
| • Get depressed and give up | • Value themselves for who they are |
| • Reach for impossible goals | • Correct mistakes, then learn from them |
| • Value themselves for what they do | • Experience disappointment but keep going |
| • Have to win to maintain high self-esteem | • Are pleased with knowing they did their best |
| • Can only live with being number one | • Enjoy meeting high standards within reach |
| • Remember mistakes and dwell on them | • Do not have to win to maintain high self-esteem |

Courtesy, White, L., Critical Thinking in Practical/Vocational Nursing, 2000, Delmar.

# EFFECTIVE USE OF AVAILABLE TIME

To plan effective use of available time, nurses must understand the big picture and decide on priority patient outcomes. No nurse works in isolation. Nurses should know what is expected of their co-workers, what is happening on the other shifts, and what is happening in the agency and the community. If the previous shift was stressed by a crisis on the unit or in the community, a shift may not get started as smoothly (Hansten & Washburn, 1998). If other hospital units outside of a nursing unit are overwhelmed, staff might be moved from one unit to assist on the overwhelmed unit elsewhere in the hospital. When nurses take the big picture into consideration, they are less likely to be frustrated when asked to assist others both on their unit and in the hospital.

## Setting Priority Patient Outcomes

Nurses set priorities to achieve safe patient outcomes. Priority setting is one of the most critical skills a nurse must develop. Nurses determine priorities by applying the nursing process, assessing the patient, and making a nursing diagnosis. The nurse then plans, implements, and evaluates patient care. This is an ongoing process, calling for constant reassessment and re-prioritization of patient care needs.

Differentiating between problems needing immediate attention and those that can wait requires great skill and judgment (Castledine, 2002). If the nurse does not prioritize care, a patient's problems may be missed and the patient's care can become even more difficult to manage. Priorities should be determined based on the patient's condition and his responses to health care problems and treatments. Being flexible in prioritizing is a key to success as a patient's status may be continuously changing.

## REAL WORLD INTERVIEW

As an emergency nurse, priorities are very important. Priorities must be flexible to change with the environment. When arriving at work, prepare by checking your patients, rooms, and equipment. Review your patients' charts and receive the Patient Report from the nurse who is going off duty. Then prioritize patient care. Priorities change when new patients arrive or a patient's condition changes. Stay ahead of the curve by anticipating what will happen during the patient's stay. For example, if a patient's problem is nausea with vomiting, I can anticipate starting the IV and collecting lab samples before the patient sees the MD. When the patient sees the MD and orders are written, the patient can then quickly receive their medicine for nausea. I take care of the patient's immediate needs and anticipate his or her future needs.

*Chris Curtis, RN, Austin, TX*

**Priority Traps.** Vacarro (2001) states that prioritizing has several traps that nurses should avoid. See Table 4-4.

A frequent prioritizing trap for nurses is the "do whatever hits first" trap. This means that a nurse may want to respond to things that the nurse sees first. For example, a nurse at the beginning of the day shift chooses to fill out the preoperative checklist for a patient going to surgery the next day before assessing the rest of the patients.

The second prioritizing trap is the "taking the path of least resistance" trap. In this trap, the nurses may make a flawed assumption that it is easier to do a task themselves rather that delegating it. For example, a nurse who is admitting a patient needs to take the patient's vital signs, weigh him, complete the baseline assessment, and call the doctor for orders. The first two tasks can be delegated to UAP so that the nurse may complete the baseline assessment of the patient and then call the doctor for orders.

The third prioritizing trap is the "responding to the squeaky wheel" trap, wherein nurses feel compelled to respond to whatever need has been vocalized the loudest. In this case, the nurse may choose to respond to a family member who has come to the nursing station every half hour with some

| TABLE 4-4 |
| :--- |
| *PRIORITIZING TRAPS TO AVOID* |
| • Doing whatever hits first |
| • Taking the path of least resistance |
| • Responding to the squeaky wheel |
| • Completing tasks by default |
| • Relying on misguided inspiration |
| Vaccaro, P. J. (April 2001). Five Priority Traps, Family Practice Management. |

concern. To appease the family, the nurse may take time to focus on one of their many verbal concerns and overlook a more pressing need elsewhere.

The fourth prioritizing trap is called the "completing tasks by default" trap. This trap occurs when nurses feel obligated to complete tasks that no one else will complete. A common example of this trap is a nurse emptying the garbage instead of asking housekeeping to do it.

The last trap is the "relying on misguided inspiration" trap. The classic example of this trap is when nurses feel 'inspired' to document findings in the chart and avoid doing a higher priority responsibility. Unfortunately, some tasks will never become inspiring and need discipline, conscientiousness, and hard work to complete them.

**Considerations in Setting Priorities.** Nurses use Maslow's Hierarchy of Needs to establish priorities. Not every patient can be seen first, even if the nurse desires to do so. For example, emergency room (ER) nurses see first priority patients immediately. Second priority urgent patients are seen quickly but they can wait a short while, usually no more than an hour or two. Third priority non-urgent patients can wait to be seen. They have no immediate threats to their Airway, Breathing, or Circulation. See Table 4-5 and 4-6.

Once nurses have decided on priority patients, they must consider what can be achieved with the available resources. Some circumstances that can deplete these resources include personnel who are late, absent, or uncooperative, or an unforeseen patient crisis. If someone has called in sick and no replacement is available, it might be unreasonable for a nurse to plan to reinforce teaching or discuss a home environment with a patient scheduled to leave the next day. However, there would be no question that interventions that prevent life-threatening emergencies or save a life when a life-threatening event occurs are priorities. They must be done no matter how short the staffing. It is a high priority that nurses protect their patients and maintain both patient and staff safety as well as perform important nursing activities.

## TABLE 4-5
### IDENTIFYING PRIORITY PATIENTS

- First Priority Emergency Patients—Remember Maslow's (1970) Hierarchy of Human Needs. Assess physiological needs first. First, examine any high priority unstable patients who have any threats to their Airway, Breathing, and Circulation (ABC's). See Table 4-6 for examples of some of these high priority patients. These patients require nursing assessment, judgment, and evaluation continuously until transfer or stabilization. Life-threatening conditions can occur at any time during the shift and may or may not be anticipated. Remember that all equipment and observations used to support and monitor the status of patients' ABCs are also a high monitoring priority, such as monitoring patient suicide threats, vital signs, level of consciousness, neurological status, skin color, temperature, pain, IV access, cardiac rhythm, oxygen, pulse oximetry, suction, urine output, and so on.

- Second Priority Urgent Patients—Assess Maslow's second level of Human Needs, i.e., safety and security next. Are there any urgent threats to patient safety and security, such as the need for fall prevention, infection control, and so on? See these patients next.

- Third Priority Non-Urgent Patients—Prioritize the patient's other needs. Patients' non-urgent needs may include love and belonging, self-esteem, and self-actualization. What does the nursing and medical plan of care include, i.e., comfort, ambulation, positioning, and so on? Stable patients who need standard, unchanging procedures with predictable outcomes are seen last.

## TABLE 4-6
### TOP PRIORITY PATIENTS WITH POTENTIAL THREATS TO THEIR AIRWAY, BREATHING, OR CIRCULATION (ABCs)

| | |
|---|---|
| Respiratory Patients | • Airway compromise<br>• Choking<br>• Asthma<br>• Chest trauma |
| Cardiovascular Patients | • Cardiac arrest<br>• Shock<br>• Hemorrhage |
| Neurological Patients | • Major head injury<br>• Unconscious<br>• Unresponsive<br>• Seizures |

(*continues*)

**Table 4-6** (*continued*)

| Other Patients | • Major trauma |
| --- | --- |
| | • Traumatic amputation |
| | • Major burn, especially if there is airway involvement |
| | • Abdominal trauma |
| | • Vaginal bleeding |
| | • Anaphylaxis |
| | • Diabetic with altered consciousness |
| | • Septic shock |
| | • Child or elder abuse |

Compiled with information from the Canadian Paediatric Triage and Acuity Scale: Implementation Guidelines for Emergency Departments. http://www.caep.ca and click on search, and enter, triage.

# STOP AND THINK

Nurses set priorities fast when they "First Look" at patients. As you approach your patient, get in the habit of observing the following:

FIRST LOOK

OVERALL
  • Airway sounds or secretions
  • Nasal flare
  • Eye contact as you approach
  • Speech
  • Interactions
  • Posture
  • Pain
  • Level of consciousness

BREATHING
  • Rate, symmetry, and depth
  • Positioning
  • Retractions

CIRCULATION
  • Color
  • Flushed
  • Cyanotic
  • Presence of IV or oxygen

(*continues*)

**Stop and Think** (*continued*)

DRAINAGE
- Urine
- Blood
- Gastric
- Stool
- Sputum

Practice your "First Look" the next time you approach a patient. Does this improve your assessment skills?

## REAL WORLD INTERVIEW

As a triage nurse, I see patients come into the Emergency Room ambulatory, by wheelchair, or on a stretcher with Emergency Medical Services (EMS). I see emergent and non-emergent patients and must set priorities. Recognizing and caring for acutely ill or injured patients is our number one priority. These include patients with asthma, chest pain, altered mental status, uncontrolled bleeding, or significant change in vital signs. These patients need to be taken back to the treatment area first. I also have to monitor the non-emergent patients and let them know they are important and will be cared for in a timely manner. Triage can be very stressful at times and keeping patients informed is very important.

*Karen Woodard, RN, Austin, Texas*

**More Priority Setting.**   Covey, Merrill, and Merrill (1994) developed another way of setting priorities. Activities are classified as:
- Urgent or not urgent
- Important or not important

If an activity is both urgent and important, it is top priority. If an activity is neither important nor urgent, then it becomes the lowest priority.

Some activities that are often thought of as important may not be. Sometimes laboratory data, vital signs, and intake and output reports are ordered to be done more frequently than the status of the patient indicates. Frequent monitoring of these parameters when a patient is stable may make no significant difference in patient outcomes. When nurses begin their shifts, they can act as a patient advocate and question the activities that make no difference in outcomes. If a nursing or medical practitioner has ordered these activities, a nurse may work to get the order changed. Nurses should give priority to the activities that they know are going to make a difference in patient outcomes. Table 4-7 can be useful in setting priorities for specific activities.

## SHIFT REPORT AND MAKING ASSIGNMENTS

When the nurse comes on duty, the shift report is given to the oncoming shift by the outgoing shift. At best, a complete report can lead to a smooth and effective start to the shift. At worst, an incomplete report can leave the on-coming shift with inadequate or old data with which to start their plan. There are several ways to deliver shift report—a face-to-face meeting, audio taping, and walking rounds. See Table 4-8.

Whether the report is conducted face-to-face, by audiotape, or through walking rounds, priority patient information has to be transmitted to allow for the effective and efficient implementation of care. If the out-going nurse fails to cover all pertinent points, the on-coming shift must ask for the appropriate information. See Table 4-9.

Nurses strive to expedite reports by focusing on major points of the patient's care and eliminating extraneous information and gossip.

**TABLE 4-7**
*PRIORITIZING ACTIVITIES*

| Urgent and Important | Urgent and Not Important | Non Urgent and Important | Non Urgent and Non Important |
|---|---|---|---|
| Take report | Patient demanding fresh cup of coffee | Specimen delivery | Socializing |
| Make rounds and assess patient needs | | Patient teaching | |
| Pass medications | | Distribute water to patients Documentation | |

Adapted from Covey, S. R., Merrill, A. R., & Merrill, R. R. (1994). First Things First: To Love, To Learn, To Leave a Legacy; NY, Simon and Schuster.

**TABLE 4-8**

**CHANGE OF SHIFT REPORTS: ADVANTAGES AND DISADVANTAGES**

### Face to Face Reports

| Advantages | Disadvantages |
|---|---|
| • Nurse giving report has actual audience and tends to be less mechanical. More likely to give pertinent information than a nurse would give to a tape recorder. | • Time consuming. It is easy to get side tracked and gossip or discuss non-patient related business. |
| • Nurses get clarification and can ask questions. | • Both oncoming and departing nurses are in report. Patients are not included in planning. |

### Audio Taped Report

| Advantages | Disadvantages |
|---|---|
| • Departing shift tapes report for oncoming shift prior to arrival of new shift workers. | • Variables in the taping process such as the quality of tape and machine, the clarity and diction of the nurse who is recording, and the hearing of the oncoming shift can interfere with the communication. |
| • Report is brief due to lack of interruptions by questions and comments | • It is difficult to get questions answered. The nurse must find a caregiver after the report to ask questions of. Information is taped earlier in the shift and may no longer be accurate. |
| • Departing shift can provide care while oncoming shift gets report. | • There is sometimes not enough information given due to the tendency of the person talking into tape recorder to read from Kardex instead of explaining about patients. |

### Walking Rounds Report

| Advantages | Disadvantages |
|---|---|
| • Provides the prior shift and oncoming shift staff the opportunity to observe the patient while receiving report. Staff can address any assessment or treatment questions. | • It is time consuming. |

*(continues)*

**Table 4-8** (*continued*)

### Walking Rounds Report

| Advantages | Disadvantages |
|---|---|
| • Departing nurse can show assessment and/or treatment data directly to oncoming nurse. | • There is a lack of privacy in discussing patient information. |
| • The patient is included in the planning and evaluation of care. The information is accurate and timely. | |
| • Accountability of outgoing care provider is promoted. | |
| • Patient views the continuity of care as oncoming shift makes initial nursing rounds with prior shift. | |

Courtesy, Maloney, P., Time Management in Kelly-Heidenthal, P. L., Nursing Leadership and Management, Delmar, 2003.

### TABLE 4-9
### *A TOOL FOR TAKING AND GIVING REPORT*

| | Information | Notes |
|---|---|---|
| Patient Data | Room number, name, sex, nursing and medical practitioner, admission date, surgery date | |
| Diagnoses and Condition | Primary and secondary nursing and medical diagnoses, current assessment of patient's condition with relevant, objective measurements —vital signs, diet, IV fluids, oxygen saturation, pain level, intake and output, skin condition, fall risk, do not | |

(*continues*)

**Table 4-9** (*continued*)

| | Information | Notes |
|---|---|---|
| Diagnoses and Condition (*continued*) | resuscitate (DNR) status, ambulation, presence or absence of signs and symptoms of potential complications, patient and family concerns, and so on. | |
| New Orders and Interventions | Any new orders, medications, labwork, or changes in treatment or teaching plan | |
| Priority Shift Outcomes and Interventions | Priority outcomes/ interventions for priority nursing and medical diagnoses, Patient learning outcomes | |
| Plans for Discharge | Expected date of discharge, any referrals needed, progress toward outcomes and self-care, readiness for home | |
| Support Needs | Availability of family or friends to assist in ADL/IADL (Activities of Daily Living/Instrumental Activities Daily Living), Problems and concerns | |

Compiled with information from Eggland and Heinemann, D. S., Nursing Documentation: Charting, Recording, and Reporting, Philadelphia, J.B. Lippincott, 1994.

# Making Assignments

During or after report, the nurse can complete an assignment sheet; a written or computerized plan that makes assignments to team members and identifies the priorities for the shift. Assignments should include specific reporting guidelines, times for interventions, and deadlines for accomplishing the tasks. Assignments should consider various factors. See Table 4-10. Note the assignment sheet excerpt in Table 4-11.

## TABLE 4-10
### *FACTORS CONSIDERED IN MAKING ASSIGNMENTS*

- Priority of patient needs
- Geography of nursing unit
- Complexity of patient need
- Other responsibilities of staff
- Attitude and dependability of staff
- Need for continuity of care by same staff
- Need for fair work distribution among staff
- Need of patient for isolation and/or protection
- Skill, education, and competency of staff, i.e., RN, LPN, UAP

## TABLE 4-11
### *ASSIGNMENT SHEET EXCERPT*

| Room, Name | Patient Description | Special Needs | Assignment |
|---|---|---|---|
| | | Take all vitals, 4 P.M. and 8 P.M. | *All to report outcomes to Mary, RN, at 8:30 P.M.—report anything abnormal STAT |
| 2501 Mr. Zagone | 25-year-old male with HIV and pneumonia, admitted last night, WBCs 3,000. TPR 100.6/ BP 126/72 | Reverse isolation, push fluids, calorie count | John, LPN |
| 2502 Mrs. Cronin | 50-year-old female, admitted yesterday with cancer of liver. Jaundiced and scheduled for port insertion today. | NPO, complaining of severe abdominal pain, hyperalimentation at 83 cc/hr. | John, LPN |
| 2503 Mrs. Thomas | 66-year-old female admitted with congestive heart failure and diabetes 3 days ago. She is on digitalis and sliding scale insulin and is noncompliant | Accuchek at 4 P.M. and 9 P.M., Up in chair with help at 6 P.M. , calorie count, teach insulin injection. | Colleen, RN |

*(continues)*

**Table 4-11** (*continued*)

| | | | |
|---|---|---|---|
| | with treatment and diet. Almost ready for discharge. | | |
| 2504 Mrs. Black | 60-year-old female transferred from ICU last night after Zoloft overdose/attempted suicide. States she wants to join her husband in heaven. | Sitter at bedside, don't leave unattended. | Colleen, RN, and Jane, sitter |

(See patient descriptions, p. xxi)

## Making Patient Care Rounds

As nurses make patient care rounds, they perform rapid assessments of each patient. The information that is gathered on rounds may change the nurse's initial plans. The nurse may get information that increases the need for patient monitoring. It is important to remember that plans are just that, plans, and need to be flexible based on ever changing patient care needs. Times for treatments and medications may have to be changed. Often nurses believe that the times for administering medications are inflexible, yet practitioners usually write medication orders to be given daily, twice a day, three times a day, or four times a day. These kinds of orders give nurses flexibility in working out administration times in cooperation with the pharmacy department, medication arrival times for computerized medication administration systems, and so on. Although unit policy dictates when these medicines are given, unit policy is under nursing control (Maloney, 2003).

## LITERATURE APPLICATION

**Citation:** Snodgrass, S. G. (2001). Wish you were a star? Become one! *Chicago Tribune,* June 10, 2001.

**Discussion:** The most logical way to predict your future is to create it, so if you want to be a star, start by becoming a top performer now. Companies are drawn to those who use up to date skills and leadership to produce measurable results. Organizations seek such people out. Surprisingly, few people understand this. You can begin to position yourself now with exceptional performance.

*(continues)*

## Literature Application (continued)

Start by delivering more than you promise and consistently outperform yourself. Exceed expectations on a regular basis; seek more responsibility; value teamwork and diversity; provide leadership and always go beyond the call of duty. Communicate effectively and know how to network with others. Be resourceful, comfortable with ambiguity, and open to saying, "I don't know but I'll find out." In addition, take initiative and persevere until you reach quantifiable results. Finally, assume some personal risk by thinking outside the box and exploring bold, new solutions to challenges. Provide yourself with a margin of confidence through life-long learning. Be open, flexible, and adapt to new ideas. Spend time with those who challenge your thinking.

You should also be creative, seek innovative solutions, and supplement your past experience with a fresh perspective. Learn how to put your ideas into action and be persistent because achieving results often takes time. In addition, do your homework. Understand the business agenda and close any gaps between what you are and what you could be. In other words, define your goals, then create and implement a personal development plan. Finally, demonstrate respect for others and apply the golden rule. Achieving great results with great behavior enables your star to rise. You can begin the process right now with these specific steps:

- See the big picture. Know why your job was created, how it relates to your organization, and what opportunities it contains. You can positively influence outcomes through performance and achievement.
- Invest in your organization; make decisions as if you owned the company. Determine which actions promise the most significant impact, and then pursue them with zeal.
- Push your comfort zone by seeking challenges, finding the positives in negative situations, taking action, and learning from the past.
- Make time for people, understand the culture, values, and beliefs of the organization, keep things in perspective, and have fun.
- Inspire those around you to exceed expectations; also, convey a sense of urgency and consistently drive issues to closure.

After you do all this, how do you ensure that you will be noticed? Ask how your company identifies and rewards top performers. Inquire as to whether or not there is a high potential category. You should pursue an environment where the best are recognized and valued. It should be an organization that provides career growth, lifelong learning, and development opportunities.

You also want meaningful work, an opportunity to contribute, and an environment that prizes new ideas and fresh perspectives. In addition, you deserve honest feedback and the opportunity to provide the same in return. Finally seek an organization that energizes and empowers you, encourages

(continues)

**Literature Application** (*continued*)

your good health, respects your point of view, and honors your performance. Many such organizations abound.

**Implications for Nursing:** Though a business professional wrote this article,
the advice rings true for nurses.

## Evaluation of Outcome Achievement

At the end of the shift, the nurse reexamines the report sheet and the assignment sheet to determine if all the assigned care was completed, the dressings
completed, labs checked, doctors notified, patient needs met, and so on. Did
the patient achieve the priority outcomes? If not, why? Were there staffing
problems or patient crises? Were the activities that were necessary for outcome
achievement carried out? Is the patient comfortable? What was learned from
this for future shifts? What will you report to the next shift?

## STOP AND THINK

Four of Steve's patients were discharged today by 10 A.M. The nursing
supervisor asked Steve to help out in the Emergency Room. Steve agreed
and was assigned to help the triage nurse. Identify the order in which
patients should be seen in the ER.

Group I
- A 2-year-old boy with chest retractions.
- A 1-year-old girl choking on a grape.
- A 5-year-old boy with a knee laceration.

You are correct if you see the 1-year-old girl choking on a grape first.
Remember your ABCs. Patients with airway problems always are seen first.
How about Group II? Which patient would you see first?

Group II
- A 60-year-old female who is nonresponsive and drooling.
- A 30-year-old male trauma patient who has absent breath sounds in
  the right side of his chest.
- A 15-year-old female who cut her wrist in an attempted suicide.

Again, the patient with the airway problem is seen first, the patient who is
nonresponsive and drooling. Of course, the patient with absent breath
sounds on one side of his chest would be seen next, and then the patient
with a cut wrist. It is best that more than one nurse is available to work with
these three patients.

## REVIEW QUESTIONS

1. General time management techniques include all except which of the following?
   A. Allowing distractions
   B. Maintaining an outcomes orientation
   C. Analyzing Time
   D. Focusing on priorities

2. Which of the following is the most efficient and effective way to give the shift report?
   A. Audio taped report
   B. Walking rounds
   C. Face-to-face meeting
   D. Any of the above

3. Personal productivity can be enhanced by:
   A. Analyzing time, getting up an hour early, and delegating unwanted tasks.
   B. Getting up an hour early, answering your phone, and inviting a friend in to talk.
   C. Analyzing use of time, getting up early, and waiting patiently.
   D. Avoiding working and going to school at the same time.

4. The nurse has just finished change of shift report. Which patient should the nurse assess first?
   A. A postoperative cholecystectomy patient who is complaining of pain but received an IM injection of Demerol (meperidine hydrochloride) five minutes ago.
   B. A postoperative appendectomy patient who will be discharged in the next few hours.
   C. A patient with asthma who had difficulty breathing during the prior shift.
   D. An elderly patient with diabetes who is on the bedpan.

5. The nurse is starting the shift at 3 P.M. Which patient should be assessed first?
   A. A new diabetic patient who received 22 units of NPH insulin at 7 A.M.
   B. A one-day post-cardiac catheterization patient.
   C. A patient who was admitted at 8:30 A.M. with abdominal pain.
   D. A patient and family awaiting discharge instructions.

6. The nurse is starting the shift at 11 P.M. What should be delegated to the UAP initially?
   A. Assessing a patient's pedal pulses that arrived on the floor at 5 p.m. post femoral popliteal graft placement.
   B. Passing fresh water to all of the patients.

    C. Taking vital signs on assigned patients prior to midnight.

    D. Turning off the IV pump alarm that is beeping.

7. The UAP asks the nurse if it would be okay to watch the nurse and learn how to do a sterile dressing change on an abdominal wound. What is the best response for the nurse?

    A. "Yes, it is good for you to learn how to do as much as you can."

    B. "Okay, but sterile dressings are only performed by licensed personnel."

    C. "I don't want you to watch as it makes me nervous."

    D. "Why do you want to help me?"

8. What task should the 3 P.M. to 11 P.M. nurse delegate to the UAP first?

    A. Restocking the linen closet.

    B. Repositioning a patient who is due to be turned.

    C. Rechecking vital signs that were elevated at noon.

    D. Transporting a patient who is to be discharged to the front door of the hospital.

9. What task may the nurse delegate to UAP?

    A. Transport a patient on a cardiac monitor to x-ray.

    B. Give tracheotomy care.

    C. Bathe stable patients.

    D. Remove sutures.

10. The nurse has initiated Cardiopulmonary Resuscitation (CPR) on a patient found on the floor. The nurse has called for help. The first person to arrive is the UAP. What will the nurse delegate to the UAP to do first?

    A. Assist with CPR.

    B. Get medications from pharmacy.

    C. Call the family and notify them of the patient's condition.

    D. Begin pushing the bed to the Intensive Care Unit (ICU).

11. The UAP reports to the nurse that a patient with a new laryngectomy is complaining of shortness of breath. What task could be delegated to the UAP by the nurse in this situation?

    A. Listen to the patient's lungs.

    B. Put the patient in Fowler's position.

    C. Suction the patient's tracheotomy tube.

    D. Change the dressing on the patient's incision.

12. The staff RN's assignment on the 7 A.M. to 3 P.M. shift includes a newly admitted patient with pneumonia who has arrived on the unit, a new post-operative surgical patient requesting pain medication, and a patient diagnosed with nephrolithiasis who is complaining of nausea. What should the nurse do first after shift report?

    A. Assess the newly admitted pneumonia patient.

    B. Give morphine to the new postoperative patient.

C. Set up the 9 A.M. medications.

D. Administer Zofran (Ondansetron hydrochloride) to the patient complaining of nausea.

13. The nurse has been assigned to a medical-surgical unit on a stormy day. Three of the staff can't make it in to work and no other staff is available. How will the nurse proceed?

    A. Prioritize care so that all patients get reasonably safe care.

    B. Provide nursing care only to those patients to whom the nurse is regularly assigned.

    C. Have the patient's family and ambulatory patients take care of the other patients.

    D. Refuse the nursing assignment as the increased number of patients makes it unsafe.

14. The nurse has just completed listening to morning report. Which patient will the nurse see first?

    A. The patient who has a leaking colostomy bag.

    B. The patient who is going for a bronchoscopy in two hours.

    C. The patient with a sickle cell crisis who has an infiltrated IV.

    D. The patient who has been receiving a blood transfusion for the last two hours and has a recent hemoglobin of 7.2 g/dl.

15. A new graduate RN who has just received her assignment asks the charge nurse, "Of the list of patients assigned to me, who do you think I should assess first?" What is the best response the charge nurse could make?

    A. "Check the policy and procedure manual for who to assess first."

    B. "Assess the patients in order of their room number to stay organized."

    C. "I would assess the patient who is having respiratory distress first."

    D. "See the patient who takes the most time last."

16. Of the following new patients, who should be assessed first by the nurse?

    A. A patient with a diagnosis of alcohol abuse with impending delirium tremens (DTs).

    B. A patient with a newly casted fractured fibula complaining of pain.

    C. A patient admitted two hours ago who is scheduled for a nephrectomy in the morning.

    D. A patient diagnosed with appendicitis that has a temperature of 100.2°F orally.

17. The nurse is making out the assignment sheet. Who is the least appropriate patient to delegate to the UAP?

    A. The patient who had a stroke and is having difficulty breathing.

    B. The patient who needs his or her blood pressure taken frequently.

    C. The patient who had heart surgery five days ago.

    D. The patient who needs to be taken for a chest x-ray.

18. The nurse has just come on duty and finished hearing morning report. Which patient will the nurse see first?
    A. The patient who is being discharged in a few hours.
    B. The patient who requires daily dressing changes.
    C. The patient who is receiving continuous IV Heparin per pump.
    D. The patient who is scheduled for an intravenous Pyelogram this shift.

19. Which patient will you delegate to the UAP?
    A. The patient who needs a daily dressing change.
    B. The patient who needs ambulation every four hours.
    C. The patient who needs a rectal suppository daily.
    D. The patient who needs teaching about diabetic diet and insulin requirements.

## REVIEW ACTIVITIES

1. Practice making assignments with the group of patients on the inside front cover of this textbook. You are the charge nurse and you have two other RNs, one unlicensed assistive personnel (UAP), and one patient sitter on the 3 P.M. to 11 P.M. shift. Your assignment sheet may look like this. See Table 4-12.

   After the first four hours of the shift had passed, the sitter, Jane, put the call light on in Room 2504. The UAP, Jill, answered the call light. Jane requested to take a 15 minute break. Jill notified Steve of the sitter's request. Nurse Steve asked Jill to see if nurse Mary could relieve the sitter. Nurse Mary was in room 2505 with a patient who was beginning to experience

### TABLE 4-12
### *MAKING ASSIGNMENTS*

| Charge nurse, Steve | RN, Colleen | RN, Mary | UAP, Jill | Sitter, Jane |
|---|---|---|---|---|
| Rooms | Rooms | Rooms | Rooms | Rooms |
| 2504 | 2508 | 2501 | 2501–2512 | 2504 |
| 2506 | 2509 | 2502 | | |
| | 2510 | 2503 | | |
| | 2511 | 2505 | | |
| | 2512 | 2507 | | |

*(continues)*

**Table 4-12** (*continued*)

| Charge responsibility, including help with all nursing and medical concerns | Total nursing care, including nursing process, orders, medications, IVs, and so on. | Total nursing care, including nursing process, orders, medications, IVs, and so on. | Complete 3–11 P.M. unit routines, including P.M. care for all patients, distribute water, answer call lights, and so on. Also, ambulate patient in room 2503 at 6 P.M.; check BP hourly on patient in room 2506; check all patient vital signs at 4 P.M. and 8 P.M.; check Glucoscan on patients in Rooms 2503 and 2511 at 4 P.M. and 9 P.M.; relieve sitter for dinner | Suicide precautions, do not leave patient unattended |
|---|---|---|---|---|

delirium tremens and nurse Colleen was checking a blood sugar on the patient with diabetes in Room 2511. Steve stated that he would not be able to leave his patient just then and Mary said she thought she could be there in a few minutes. The UAP reported back to nurse Steve the status of the situation. In the meantime the ER was on the phone ready to give report on a patient with Chronic Obstructive Pulmonary Disease (COPD). Nurse Steve told the UAP, Jill, to keep an eye on the patient in 2504 while the sitter went on break. Fifteen minutes later, the sitter, Jane, returned to room 2504. She began to scream and yelled for help. The patient had hung herself with her sheets. Nurse Steve asked the UAP, "Jill, how could this have happened? I told you to keep an eye on the patient." Jill replied, "I kept checking in on her." Nurse Steve yelled, "Checking in on her, you were not to leave her alone!"

Was the UAP delegated a duty that was within her scope of practice? How would you have handled this situation when the sitter asked for a break?

2. You go to work one day and there are too many staff on the unit. Several patients have been discharged. The nursing supervisor asks you to float to another medical surgical unit. Note the example of the use of priority setting in caring for a group of three patients on this unit. See Table 4-13.

**TABLE 4-13**
*PRIORITY ASSESSMENTS, GROUP I*

| Patient | Priority Nursing Assessments |
| --- | --- |
| Ms. JD is a 68-year-old who is post-op day 1 after a total shoulder replacement following a traumatic fall. She is confused and on multiple medications with a history of hypertension and multiple falls. She is anxious and frightened by the "visiting spirits." Her daughter stays with her at all times. | Vital signs, safety, distal pulse, incision/dressing check, and breath sounds. See this patient third during rounds. Safety is a prime concern with this confused patient as well as watching for any post operative concerns. |
| Mr. DB is a 35-year-old with insulin-dependent diabetes mellitus, juvenile onset at age twelve. He is post-op day 2 after a right below-the-knee amputation. He complains of severe right leg pain and is restless. Mr. DB has a history of non-compliance with diet and is on sliding scale insulin administration. | Vital signs, Glucoscan at 4 P.M. and 9 P.M., safety, incision/dressing check, pain, DB teaching. See this patient second during rounds. He has pain, restlessness, and a relatively new amputation. He is a diabetic and could be having a post operative complication or an insulin reaction. Evaluate restlessness carefully. |

*(continues)*

**Table 4-13** (*continued*)

| Patient | Priority Nursing Assessments |
| --- | --- |
| Mr. JK is a 35-year-old patient with a history of alcohol abuse admitted for severe abdominal pain. He is throwing up coffee-ground-like emesis. | Level of consciousness, seizure and shock potential, hematemesis, DTs, safety, vital signs, CBC, hematocrit, type & cross-match, 16-gauge IV line, oxygen, cardiac monitor. See this patient first during rounds. He is a candidate for the development of shock and DT's. |

Now, identify the priority nursing assessments for this next group of patients back on your regular unit. See Table 4-14.

**TABLE 4-14**
*PRIORITY ASSESSMENTS, GROUP II*

| Patient | Priority Nursing Assessments |
| --- | --- |
| Mrs. Homan, a 61-year-old with a hypertensive crisis three days ago, blood pressure decreasing daily, now 180/102. She periodically complains of headache. | |
| Mrs. Glusak, a 67-year-old transferred two hours ago from ICU with a recent brain attack/CVA, non-responsive, and has right sided paralysis. Family at bedside. | |
| Mrs. Zurich, a 78-year-old with cellulitis of the right toe and a history of diabetes mellitus, needs teaching. | |
| (See patient descriptions, pp. xxi–xxii) | |

3. The charge nurse on a 12-bed adult unit assigned each nurse four patients. Colleen, R.N., has just finished her five month orientation period on the unit. The charge nurse asked Colleen how she felt about coming off orientation today. Colleen stated "I am comfortable with the procedures, routines, and doctor interactions. I am still having trouble prioritizing what I should do first." The charge nurse assured her that her lack of experience

probably had a lot to do with her difficulty prioritizing. The charge nurse went to her locker and gave Colleen a handy little prioritizing chart the charge nurse has had since she graduated from nursing school. She told Colleen that she found this quick little reference chart helped her in situations when she was unsure of priorities. Colleen was grateful for the chart and she used it that day.

Colleen was assigned three patients. Mrs. Glusak, Room 2509, is a 67-year-old female, transferred two hours ago from ICU with a CVA. She is non-responsive and has right-sided paralysis. Her family is at her bedside. Colleen also has Mr. Olson, an 89-year-old male, admitted yesterday with renal failure who is confused at times and will be dialyzed soon. She also has Mrs. Zurich, a 78-year-old female, admitted with diabetes and cellulitis of the right toe, who needs teaching. Use this priority chart to determine whom Colleen will see first. See Table 4-15.

Based on the total points, Mrs. Glusak, the patient with the CVA needs to be assessed by Colleen first. Based on the priority chart, Mr. Olson, the patient with the renal failure should be assessed next.

Were you torn between the patient with a CVA and the patient who was confused? Remember, you need to assess Mrs. Glusak's airway first since the stroke left her non-responsive. Then assure Mr. Olson's safety quickly. Remember that a nurse must assess the ABCs first.

**TABLE 4-15**
*PRIORITY CHART*

| Patient's Diagnosis | Maslow's Hierarchy of Needs: 1—Physiological 2—Safety 3—Love and Belonging, Self Esteem, Self Actualization | Priority: 1—Emergency 2—Urgent 3—Non urgent | Total: The patient with the lowest total score is seen first by the nurse |
| --- | --- | --- | --- |
| Mrs. Glusak, Recent CVA | 1 | 2 | 3 |
| Mr. Olson, Renal Failure | 2 | 2 | 4 |
| Mrs. Zurich, Diabetic Cellulitis | 3 | 3 | 6 |

4. For the next three days complete an activity log for both your personal time and your work time. On what activities are you spending the majority of time? When is your energy level the highest? Is your energy level related to food intake? What are your biggest time wasters? How can you schedule your time more productively?

5. Even the simplest priority setting can make a difference in the plan of care for a group of patients. Mary, the 3 P.M. to 11 P.M. nurse received report on her group of five patients with a possible admission from the emergency room. Mary prioritized her plan of care. First she would assess the five patients, second, administer scheduled/prn medications, and then start documentation of the care she had given so far. As soon as the cafeteria opened, around 4:30 P.M., she would eat her dinner. It would be an early dinner but if she did not eat then, the chance of her getting to the cafeteria after the patient arrived from the emergency room would be low. Admitting a patient sometimes takes up to two hours to complete. Mary would get very hungry if she did not get a chance to go to the cafeteria when it was open. Taking care of oneself will benefit the patients as well. How do you prioritize and plan your clinical care? Do you take care of meeting your own needs as well as your patients?

## EXPLORING THE WEB

1. Access the site for the Canadian Association of Emergency Physicians. Note the Pediatric Triage Scale.
   http://www.caep.ca/click on search/
   Search for TRIAGE.

2. If you would like to find a system for managing your time, the following web sites offer electronic organizers, e.g., Casio electronic organizer, Sharp electronic organizer, Palm Pilot electronic organizer.
   (http://www.casio.com)
   (http:// www.sharp-usa.com)
   (http://www.palm.com)
   If you prefer a less technological time management system, the following web sites offer non-electronic organizers and systems for time management, e.g., Day timer, Covey, Franklin.
   (http://www.daytimers.com)
   (http://www.covey.com)
   (http://www.franklin.com)
   Find a free on-line calendar that you can access from anywhere.
   (http://calendar.yahoo.com)

Look at all the hints and free tools on time management at the Mind Tools web site. Can you put any of the ideas to use? (http://www. mindtools. com)

If you find time management an impossible challenge, you can find professional assistance at the Professional Organizers web site. (http://www. organizerswebring.com/)

Check out this University of Michigan site for time management tips. (http://www.umich.edu. Search for Stress Manager)

## REFERENCES

Burke, T. A., McKee, J. R., Wilson, H. C., Donahue, R. M., Batenhorst, A. S., & Pathak, D. S. (2000). A comparison of time-and-motion and self-reporting methods of work measurement. *Journal of Nursing Administration, 30*(3), 118–125.

Canadian Paediatric Triage and Acuity Scale (n.d.). *Implementation Guidelines for Emergency Departments.* http://www.caep.ca/Search for Triage.

Castledine, G. (2002). Prioritizing care is an essential nursing skill. *British Journal of Nursing, 11*(14), 987.

Covey, S. R., Merrill, A. R., & Merrill, R. R. (1994). *First things first: to love, to learn, to leave a legacy.* New York, NY: Simon & Schuster.

Eggland, E. T., & Heinemann, D. S. (1994). *Nursing documentation: Charting, recording, and reporting.* Philadelphia: J.B. Lippincott.

Fryxell, D. A. (1997). The 80% solution. *Writer's Digest, 77*(5), 57.

Graham, A. (1998). The vital few, the trivial many. *Internal Auditor, 55*(6), 6.

Grohar-Murray, M. E., & DiCroce, H. R. (1997). Managing resources. In *Leadership and management in nursing* (pp. 291–315). Stanford, CT: Appleton & Lange.

Hansten, R. I., & Washburn, M. J. (1998). *Clinical delegation skills: A handbook for professional practice.* Gaithersburg, MD: Aspen Publications.

Koch, R. (1999). *The 80/20 principle: The secret to success by achieving more with less.* New York, NY: Doubleday.

Maloney, P. L. (2003). Time management. In P. Kelly-Heidenthal, *Nursing leadership and management.* Clifton Park, New York: Delmar.

Maslow, A. H. (1970). *New knowledge in human values.* Washington, DC: Regnery Publishing, Inc., an Eagle Publishing Company.

*Mind tools: How to achieve more with your time.* (1995–1998). Retrieved Sept 5, 2000, from http://www.mindtools.com/tmintro.html.

*Mind tools: How to achieve more with your time.* (1995–1998). Retrieved Sept 5, 2000, from http://www.mindtools.com/tmgetup.html.

Prescott, P. A. Phillips, C. Y., Ryan, J. W., & Thompson, K. O. (1991). Changing how nurses spend their time. *Image Journal of Nursing Scholarship, 23*(1), 23–28.

Reed, F. C., & Pettigrew, A. C. (1999). Self-management: stress and time. In P. S. Yoder-Wise (Ed.). *Leading and managing in nursing* (2nd ed., pp. 185–204). St. Louis, MO: Mosby.

Snodgrass, S.G. (2001). Wish you were a star? Become one! *Chicago Tribune,* June 10, 2001.

Sullivan, E. J., & Decker, P. J. (1997). Stress and time management. In *Effective leadership and management in nursing* (4th ed., pp. 215–232). Menlo Park, CA: Addison-Wesley.

Scharf, L. (1997). Revising nursing documentation to meet patient outcomes. *Nursing Management 28*(4), 38–39.

Upenieks, V. B. (1998). Work sampling: Assessing nursing efficiency. *Nursing Management, 49*(4), 27–29.

Urden, L., & Roode, J. (1997). Work sampling: A decision-making tool for determining resources and work redesign. *Journal of Nursing Administration, 27*(9), 34–41.

Vacarro, P. J. (April 2001). Five priority-setting traps. *Family Practice Management, 8*(4), 60.

White, L. (2002). *Critical thinking in practical/vocational nursing.* Albany, NY: Delmar.

## SUGGESTED READINGS

Anderson, L. A. (2001). Reality research: project time management and recruitment. *Journal of Vascular Nursing 19*(4), 137–138.

Dawes, B. S. (1999). Perspectives on priorities, time management, and patient care. *Association of Perioperative Registered Nurses Journal, 70*(3), 374, 376–377.

Duffy, B. (1999). Organizing thoughts about time management. *Home Healthcare Nurse Manager, 3*(6), 14–17.

Hindle, T. (1999). *Essential managers: Manage your time.* London: DK Publishing.

Morgenstern, Julie. (2000). *Time management from the inside out: The foolproof system for taking control of your schedule and your life.* New York, NY: Henry Holt & Company.

# CHAPTER 5

Every act whatever of man that causes damage to another obliges him whose fault it happened to repair it. . . .

(LA Civil Code Article 2315)

# Legal Aspects of Patient Care and Delegation

## OBJECTIVES

*Upon completion of this chapter, the reader should be able to:*

1. Identify selected torts.

2. Discuss negligence and malpractice.

3. Discuss malpractice cases reported in the Professional Negligence Law Reports, July 2001 through July 2002.

4. Discuss clinical settings of malpractice cases.

5. Describe health care facility liabilities other than nursing actions.

6. Identify resources for safe, legal, and ethical nursing practice.

7. Review nursing risk in litigation.

8. Discuss a nursing checklist to decrease risk of liability.

9. Describe common monetary awards in malpractice cases.

10. Discuss the nurse attorney relationship in a lawsuit.

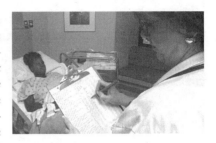

*Colleen, RN, is busy with the four patients in Rooms 2509 through 2512. Colleen receives a new intravenous piggyback (IVPB) medication order from the practitioner and orders it from the pharmacy for Mrs. Glusak, the patient in Room 2509. When the unit clerk tells Colleen that her patient's IVPB medication has arrived from the pharmacy, Colleen quickly grabs the medication and hangs it. A few minutes later, the patient becomes short of breath. As Colleen checks over her patient, she notes to her horror that she hung another patient's IVPB for this patient. What action should Colleen take immediately? What should Colleen do next? What should she do to prevent future errors? What should the hospital pharmacy and the nursing unit do to prevent future errors? Is a problem like this the fault of the system or the fault of the nurse or both?*

(See patient descriptions, p. xxii)

L aw that affects the relationship between individuals is called **civil law.** Most legal cases involving nurses fall into the category of civil tort law (Fiesta, 1999). Law that specifies the relationship between citizens and the state is called public law. This chapter reviews selected torts and common areas of nursing malpractice. It identifies actions a nurse can take to minimize risks to professional practice. It also identifies a nursing checklist to decrease the risk of liability, common monetary awards in malpractice cases, and the nurse attorney relationship in a lawsuit.

## TORT LAW

*Black's Law Dictionary* (2001) defines **tort** as a private or civil wrong or injury, including action for bad faith breach of contract, for which the court will provide a remedy in the form of an action for damages. A tort can be any of the following:

1. The denial of a person's legal right,
2. The failure to comply with a public duty, or
3. The failure to perform a private duty that results in harm to another.

A tort can be unintentional, as occurs in malpractice or neglect. It can also be the intentional infliction of harm such as assault and battery. In a tort suit, the nurse can be named as a defendant because of something the nurse did incorrectly or because the nurse failed to do something that was required. In either case, the suit is usually classified as a tort suit. Other tort charges that a nurse may face include assault and battery, false imprisonment, invasion of privacy, and defamation. See Table 5-1.

Nurses must take care to avoid these torts both when they consider nursing action themselves and when they delegate nursing actions to others.

# Negligence and Malpractice

If a nurse fails to meet the legal expectations for care, usually defined by the state's nurse practice act, the patient harmed by this failure can initiate an action against the nurse for damages inflicted either by the nurse personally or for damages inflicted by others to whom the nurse has delegated care. **Negligence** is the failure to provide the care a reasonable person would ordinarily

### TABLE 5-1
### *SELECTED TORTS*

| Tort | Definition | Example |
|---|---|---|
| Assault | Threat to touch another person in an offensive manner without that person's permission | Nurse who threatens to give a patient a treatment against his will |
| Battery | Touching of another person without that person's consent | Nurse who forces a treatment against a patient's will |
| Invasion of Privacy | All patients have the right to privacy and may bring charges against any person who violates this right | Nurse who tells information about a patient or photographs a patient without consent |
| False Imprisonment | Restriction of the freedom of an individual | Nurse who restrains a patient who is of sound mind and is not in danger of injuring himself or others |
| Defamation, including libel and slander | Intentionally false communication or publication, including written (libel) or verbal (slander) remarks that may cause the loss of a person's reputation | Nurse who makes a statement that could either ruin the patient's reputation or cause the patient to lose his job |

provide in a similar situation. The term **malpractice** refers to a professional's wrongful conduct in discharge of their professional duties or failure to meet standards of care for the profession which results in harm to another individual entrusted to the nurse's care. (Zerwekh & Claborn, 2002).

Simply proving negligence or malpractice is not sufficient to recover damages. Proof of liability or fault requires proof of the following four elements:

1. A duty or obligation created by law, contract, or standard practice that is owed to the complainant by the professional.
2. A breach of this duty, either by omission or commission.
3. Harm, which can be physical, emotional or financial, to the complainant (patient).
4. Proof that the breach of duty caused the complained of harm.

A Louisiana appellate court recently described the plaintiff patient's specific burden of proof in a negligence or malpractice case against a nurse as:

> [T]he three requirements which a plaintiff must satisfy to meet its burden of proving the negligence of a nurse: (1) the nurse must exercise the degree of skill ordinarily employed, under similar circumstances, by the members of the nursing or health care profession in good standing in the same community or locality; (2) the nurse either lacked this degree of knowledge or skill or failed to use reasonable care and diligence, along with her best judgment in the application of that skill; and (3) as a proximate result of this lack of knowledge or skill or the failure to exercise this degree of care, the plaintiff suffered injuries that would not, otherwise have occurred. (*Odom v. State Dept. of Health and Hospitals,* 1999).

Once a plaintiff presents his or her case, the defendant nurse must show either that if a duty was owed, it was fulfilled, or the nurse must show that the breach of that duty was not the cause of the plaintiff's harm. This must be demonstrated for care delivered by the nurse personally and for care delegated by the nurse to others.

Proving that a duty was owed is not difficult. The person need only show that the nurse was working on the day in question and was responsible either for the plaintiff's care personally or for delegating the plaintiff's care to others. This can usually be accomplished by producing staffing schedules, assignment sheets, job descriptions, policies on delegation, and so on.

To demonstrate a breach of duty, the courts employ a reasonable man standard. The test applied for determining this standard is, what would a reasonable and prudent nurse do under the same or similar circumstances? The standard is illustrated by reviewing such documents as the employing institution's policies and procedures, the state nurse practice act, the National Council of State Boards of Nursing (NCSBN) Delegation Decision-Making

Grid, the Joint Commission on Accreditation of Health Care Organizations' Standards, and by hearing testimony from nurses who are accepted as expert witnesses to the standard of nursing practice in the community. What is "reasonable and prudent care" can be determined from a variety of sources. See Table 5-2.

The defendant nurse would employ the same methodology to refute the plaintiff's charges. The nurse would present evidence that the institution's policies and procedures were followed and that the care rendered adhered to accepted nursing standards. To present the nurse's case, the nurse's attorney would also use expert witnesses to document that the care given or delegated fulfilled the duty owed, was the kind that would be given or delegated by a reasonable nurse in such a circumstance, and that it was not the cause of the plaintiff's harm.

It is not sufficient for a patient plaintiff to show a breach of duty to prevail in a tort suit. He must also show that the breach of the duty caused him harm. Even if it is proven that a nurse made a medication error or delegated this action incorrectly, if the error was not the cause of the plaintiff's harm, the plaintiff will not win in recovering damages from the nurse. In a recent malpractice case, a patient with sickle cell anemia died after suffering a cardio-pulmonary arrest, attributed to an aspiration that was witnessed by a visitor. The visitor immediately called for and obtained help. Although revived, the patient never regained consciousness and was eventually taken off life-support. At trial

## TABLE 5-2
### SOURCES OF EVIDENCE REGARDING A STANDARD OF CARE

- Evidence-Based Health Care Literature
- Nursing and Medical Textbooks, Articles, and Research
- State Professional Practice Acts, i.e., Nurse Practice Act, Physician Practice Act
- Standards of Professional Association, e.g., American Nurses' Association Standards
- Equipment Manufacturers Manuals, e.g., Cardiac Monitoring Equipment Manuals
- Written Policies and Procedures of a Facility, e.g., Foley Catheter Insertion Procedures
- Nurse, Physician, or other Health Care Professional Expert Testimony
- Professional Health Care Accreditation Agency Criteria, e.g., JCAHO Criteria
- Medication Books, e.g., *Physician's Desk Reference, American Society of Health System Pharmacists Drug Information Book,* and so on.

the plaintiff's attorney was able to prove that the nurse assigned to this patient did not follow the institution's policies in documenting the frequent observations needed because the patient was receiving a blood transfusion at the time of the cardiac arrest. In reviewing the case on appeal, the appellate court noted:

> [T]he record contains no evidence which suggests what could have been done even if the nurse had been seated at his bedside prior to the arrest. Plaintiff has failed to offer any proof that more immediate assistance would have prevented the catastrophic results of his aspiration. Based on the evidence in this record, we conclude that more frequent monitoring would have made no difference. *Webb v Tulane Medical Center Hospital,* 700 So.2d. 1141,1145 (4th Cir. 1997).

Thus, even though the plaintiff successfully proved a breach of a duty, the breach was not found to be the cause of the patient's death and the nurse was not found to be guilty of negligence. See Table 5-3 for the types of nursing malpractice cases reported in the Professional Negligence Law Reporter from July 2001 through July 2002. Table 5-4 discusses the clinical settings of these nursing malpractice cases. Table 5-5 discusses health care facility liabilities other than nursing actions.

When a nurse is listed as a party in a malpractice lawsuit, the nurse's liability is determined by state laws, such as the nurse practice act, the standards for the practice of nursing, and the institution's policies and procedures. Thus, if the laws mandate that a nurse must have a doctor's order before doing something, then the doctor's order must be present. Problems arise when the orders are verbal, and later, it is claimed that the nurse misunderstood and acted in error. To prevent this type of malpractice, nurses have adopted the practice of repeating all verbal and phone orders back to the practitioner after receiving them and documenting this practice. See Chapter 3. Another pitfall is illegible writing, which is then misinterpreted and the result causes harm to the patient.

Nurses who have been in practice for a long time have encountered nursing and medical practitioners who write orders that are contrary to accepted practice. In these situations, the nurse must exercise professional judgment and follow the policies and procedures of the institution. Usually these require the nurse to clarify the order with the practitioner and discuss the order as needed with the nursing supervisor and the medical director for the area in which the nurse works in order to clarify it (Martin & Cain, 2003).

As mentioned earlier, practicing nurses must also adhere to the standards for practice for the nursing profession in the community. These standards include such things as checking the six "rights" of medication administration (the right patient, medication, dose, time, route, and documentation), and

## TABLE 5-3
### *NURSING MALPRACTICE CASES**

- Failed to prevent and treat pressure ulcers and malnutrition resulting in death[5]
- Mishandled shoulder dystocia during delivery resulting in brachial plexus injury[6]
- Failed to perform intrauterine resuscitation leading to infant's brain damage[11]
- Failed to properly handle telephone triage calls resulting in death[12]
- Failed to incorporate patient's emergency room records into patient's hospital chart resulting in death[12]
- Failed to properly treat pediatric glaucoma resulting in vision loss[13]
- Burned patient with hair dryer resulting in third-degree burns[15]
- Failed to accurately count sponges after operation resulting in retained sponge[16]
- Failed to provide adequate nutrition and implement nursing plan of care resulting in death[19]
- Injected patient with used needle leading to emotional distress from possible hepatitis infection[23]
- Failed to properly treat patient's jaundice resulting in infant's brain damage[24]
- Failed to treat dehydration and pressure ulcers resulting in death[27]
- Removed internal pacemaker wires improperly resulting in infection[29]
- Administered suction tube improperly, leading to aspiration and death by suffocation[30]
- Failed to detect arterial blockage after surgery leading to leg amputation[32]
- Failed to adequately hydrate patient prior to Cesarean delivery resulting in maternal hypotension and infant's brain damage[33]
- Failed to administer supplemental oxygen resulting in vision loss and brain damage[44]

### Communication

- Failed to notify physician of
  a. patient burns[15]
  b. bleeding gastric ulcer, resulting in death[9]
  c. increased heart rate, resulting in death[14]
  d. fetal distress, resulting in death[3] resulting in brain damage [17,22]
  e. newborn jaundice, resulting in brain damage[24]
  f. PT level[29]
  g. pain and numbness after spinal surgery, resulting in cauda equina syndrome[39]
  h. vision problems, resulting in vision loss[40]
- Failed to report sexual abuse of patient/ resident to police and/or state department of human resources[10,31]

*(continues)*

**Table 5-3** (*continued*)

• Failed to institute chain of command when physician refused to come to the hospital promptly[26][37]

## Medication

• Administered insufficient Heparin, leading to death by pulmonary embolism[1]
• Administered doses of Dilantin and insulin to a patient in excess of physician's order, leading to patient's disorientation and burns by bedside heater[4]
• Administered excessive dose of IV antibiotics (Nafcillin) leading to chemical burn[18]
• Failed to send antibiotics home with patient with meningitis, leading to cerebral palsy[28]
• Failed to recognize dosage error in doctor's order and thereby administered excessive dose of Dilaudid, leading to brain damage[36]

## Monitoring/ Observing/ Supervising

• Failed to monitor premature newborn, leading to death by cardiac arrest[2]
• Failed to detect fetal distress, resulting in death[3] resulting in brain damage [17][22][46][47]
• Failed to monitor patient, leading to third degree burns[4]
• Failed to timely call a "code blue" in response to patient's respiratory arrest, resulting in death[7]
• Failed to prevent patient falls, leading to death[8] leading to quadriplegia [42] leading to quadriparesis[43]
• Failed to seek timely medical intervention, leading to death from bleeding ulcer[9]
• Failed to properly monitor heart rate after surgery, resulting in death[14]
• Misidentified and mixed up newborns in nursery[20]
• Failed to monitor respiratory rate after surgery, resulting in death[21]
• Failed to take vital signs of patient in waiting room, resulting in brain damage[34]
• Failed to restrain demented patient, resulting in death[35]
• Failed to properly insert foley catheter during delivery, resulting in urinary sphincter trauma and incontinence[38]
• Failed to monitor cornea in facial palsy, leading to corneal scarring and vision loss[40]
• Failed to reattach cardiac monitor after x-rays, resulting in death[41]
• Failed to detect brain swelling, resulting in vision loss and diminished I.Q.[45]

*Reported in Professional Negligence Law Reporter, July 2001 through July 2002 (Courtesy, Pozza, R., Unpublished manuscript, 2003)

## TABLE 5-4
### CLINICAL SETTINGS OF NURSING MALPRACTICE CASES *

| Clinical Setting | No. of Cases |
|---|---|
| Hospital-Medical-Surgical [7 15 16 18 21 25 29 32 36 39 40 43 45] | 13 |
| Maternity-Obstetrics [3 6 11 17 22 26 33 38 46 47] | 10 |
| Nursing Home [4 5 8 9 19 27 30 31 35] | 9 |
| Emergency Room [1 12 23 41 42] | 5 |
| Pediatrics-Nursery [2 20 24 28] | 4 |
| Recovery Room [14 37] | 2 |
| Home Health Care [10 44] | 2 |
| Clinic [13] | 1 |
| Urgent Care Facility [34] | 1 |
| **Total** | **47** |

*Reported in Professional Negligence Law Reporter, July 2001 through July 2002 (Courtesy, Pozza, R., Unpublished manuscript, 2004)

## TABLE 5-5
### HEALTH CARE FACILITY LIABILITIES OTHER THAN NURSING ACTIONS*

- Failure to provide a safe environment[4 30 35]
- Misrepresenting level of care available at nursing home[5]
- Failure to adequately train personnel in fall prevention[8]
- Failure to adequately supervise nursing home staff to ensure residents received proper nutrition, custodial treatment, and medical care[19]
- Failure to instruct and train personnel regarding the handling of jaundice in newborns[24]
- Failure to adequately train staff on emergency procedures[34]
- Failure to inform physician of patient burns[15]
- Failure to properly supervise staff[10 19]
- Failure to provide timely lab services[23]
- Failure to appropriately dispose of used syringes[23]
- Failure to enforce policies to adequately handle emergencies[30]
- Failure to report abuse of nursing home resident[31]
- Allowing unlicensed persons to administer IV medications[34]

*Reported in Professional Negligence Law Reporter, July 2001 through July 2002 (Courtesy, Pozza, R., Unpublished manuscript, 2003)

using the concepts of the NCSBN Delegation Decision-Making Grid in making assignments. See Chapter 2. It is not uncommon for the nurse to find conflicts between an employer's expectations and nursing standards of care. This results in problems such as having insufficient time or staffing to adhere to the standards taught in nursing school or receiving poor evaluations for taking too long to deliver care. In these situations, the nurse must identify what standards to follow to preserve professional nursing practice, to protect patients, and to keep the nurse from liability. Maintaining clear communication with nursing and medical practitioners and the supervisors that one works with helps to limit the nurse's exposure to liability.

## Do Not Attempt to Resuscitate (DNAR) Orders and Following Orders

The attending physician may write a Do Not Attempt to Resuscitate (DNAR) order on a patient, which directs the staff not to perform the usual cardiopulmonary resuscitation (CPR) in the event of a sudden cardiopulmonary arrest. The doctor may write such an order without evidence of a living will on the medical record and the nurse should be familiar with the institution's policies and state law regarding when and how a physician can write such an order in the absence of a living will. Often, a DNAR order is considered a medical decision that the doctor can make, preferably in consultation with the family, even without an executed living will by the patient.

If the nurse feels that a DNAR order or any order is contrary to the patient's good, the nurse should consult the policies and procedure of the institution. As identified in Chapter 1, these policies include going up the administrative chain of command until the nurse is satisfied with the course of action and has assured patient safety. This may entail notifying the physician, other nursing and medical practitioners, the charge nurse, the nursing supervisor, the nursing director, the medical director, the risk manager, the institution's Chief Operating Officer, state regulators, and/or The Joint Commission on Accreditation of Health Care Organizations (JCAHO). Often an institution has an ethics committee that may examine such issues and make a determination of the appropriateness of the order.

## REAL WORLD INTERVIEW

I took care of a postoperative patient who developed a wound infection when his incision did not heal after a wound dehiscence that was left open to heal on its own. I worked with this patient's doctor on a regular basis on the unit where I was assigned. The doctor told me that he was just going to watch the patient for a while as he thought the wound dehiscence would

*(continues)*

**Real World Interview** (*continued*)

heal by itself. This did not happen and I lost faith in the physician as the patient was doing poorly. I talked again with the patient's doctor who continued to say that he was just going to watch it. I mentioned to him that I was concerned about the patient and was going to discuss my concerns with the supervisor, hoping he would respond to this gentle nudge and take the initiative and do something more for the patient. I had worked with this doctor for a long time. When he did not take any action, I reported my concerns to my supervisor. The supervisor reported the situation to the Director of Nursing who discussed the case with the Chief of the Medical Staff. The Chief of the Medical Staff then discussed the case with the original doctor who agreed to ask another surgeon for a consultation. They did this and took the patient back to surgery. While I was happy for the patient who did well, I felt bad about my relationship with the original doctor who I continued to work with daily. He never spoke to me again. I know I did the right thing. I wish it were easier.

*Patricia Kelly-Heidenthal*, RN

# RESOURCES FOR SAFE, LEGAL, AND ETHICAL NURSING PRACTICE

There are many resources that assist nurses in determining what is safe nursing practice. Nurses should be familiar with these in performing their duties. A few key resources are discussed here.

## State Nurse Practice Act

The nurse practice act in each state specifies the legal parameters of nursing practice in that state. It answers questions regarding what a nurse can legally do in that state and this may vary from state to state. The nurse must know what a nurse is allowed to do in the state where he or she practices. It is not sufficient to say, "I know how to do this and I was allowed to do it in Nebraska." If a practice is not within the scope of nursing as it is defined in Mississippi, the nurse cannot do it in Mississippi. To find access to state boards of nursing contact the web site www.ncsbn.org.

## Policies and Procedures of the Institution

In most conflicts regarding nursing care, the institution's policies and procedures are examined and are usually admitted as evidence of what the nurse is expected to do. Failure to follow the policies and procedures of the institution in providing care can expose the nurse to personal liability without the protection of the institution. Nurses must know the policies and procedures of their employers and adhere to these in everyday practice.

## Good Samaritan Laws

**Good Samaritan Laws** are laws that have been enacted to protect the health care professional from legal liability for actions rendered in an emergency when the professional is giving service without pay. The essential elements of the commonly enacted Good Samaritan Law are:

1. The care is rendered in an emergency situation,
2. The health care worker is rendering care without pay, and
3. The care provided did not recklessly or intentionally cause injury or harm to the injured party.

Note that Good Samaritan laws are intended to protect the volunteer who stops to render care at the scene of an accident. They would not protect a nurse, Emergency Medical Technician (EMT), or other health care professional rendering care at the scene of an accident as part of their assigned duties and for which they receive pay. These paid emergency personnel would be evaluated according to the standards of their professions in doing their duties (Martin & Cain, 2003).

## Good Communication

The nurse must communicate accurately and completely both verbally and in writing. Many lawsuits result from a lack of communication by the nurse or other health care providers. Either the nurse failed to monitor the patient and notify the nursing or medical practitioner of a change in the patient's status; or the nurse failed to document assessments performed or failed to demonstrate competent caring nursing practice to the patient. It is essential that the nurse communicates thoughtfully with the patient and charts accurately and completely. Patients are less likely to sue if they feel that a nurse has been caring and professional. Often a case involving patient care takes several years to come to trial. By that time, the nurse may have no memory of the incident in question and must rely on the written record done at the time of the incident. This record is frequently in the courtroom, blown up to billboard size for all to see. All errors are apparent and omissions stand out by their absence, especially if it is something that should have been recorded per the institution's policy. The old adage that if it isn't documented, it isn't done, will be repeated to the jury numerous times.

Most nurses are familiar with the phrase, "If it was not documented, it was not done." Insofar as this phrase is used to encourage thorough documentation, it reflects good nursing practice. Timely, accurate, and complete documentation is an excellent way to protect oneself from litigation. However, lawyers who represent plaintiffs in medical malpractice cases are aware of this "rule" and often attempt to use it against nurses in health care liability claims.

Imagine the following scenario: A patient is admitted to the hospital and Nurse A performs an initial assessment of the patient. Nurse A notes in the patient's chart that the patient has good capillary refill. Nurse A proceeds to take the patient's vital signs, including capillary refill, hourly throughout Nurse A's 8-hour shift. The patient's capillary refill remains good and the nurse makes no further documentation in the chart relating to the patient's capillary refill. After Nurse A's shift, Nurse B takes over the patient's care. One hour into Nurse B's shift, the patient codes and expires. The patient's family sues Nurse A. The plaintiffs' lawyer is cross-examining Nurse A.

Lawyer: "Nurse A, are you familiar with the phrase, 'If it wasn't documented, it wasn't done'?"

Nurse A: "Yes."

Lawyer: "That's a common rule in nursing practice, isn't it?"

Nurse A: "Yes."

Lawyer: "You were taught that in nursing school, weren't you?"

Nurse A: "Yes, I was."

Lawyer: "And after you documented that the patient had good capillary refill upon admission, you did not document anything relating to the patient's capillary refill for the next eight hours, did you?"

Nurse A: "Well, no."

Lawyer: "So if we use your rule, 'If it wasn't documented, it wasn't done' we can assume you never checked the patient's capillary refills during your shift after the initial assessment, right?"

Nurse A: "No. I checked, but it hadn't changed, so I didn't document anything . . ."

Notice what just happened in the above exchange. Nurse A provided competent nursing care, but the lawyer made it appear as if Nurse A was negligent. A nurse involved in litigation should not blanketly agree with the documentation rule. You simply cannot document everything noted in an assessment of a patient. Moreover, most nurses would agree that patient care takes priority over documentation. This rule ignores that. Bad documentation looks bad. Good documentation protects you. Even lapses in documentation do not correlate with bad nursing care. Nurses should not lose sight of that when faced with litigation.

*Robyn D. Pozza, JD*
*Austin, Texas*

## LITERATURE APPLICATION

**Citation:** Croke, E. M. (2003). Nurses, negligence, and malpractice. *American Journal of Nursing, 103*(9), 54–64.

**Discussion:** This article discusses the actions that prompted charges of negligence that led to malpractice lawsuits against nurses from 1995 to 2001. It identifies several factors that have contributed to the increase in malpractice cases against nurses. According to the National Practitioner Data Bank (NPDB), 2,311 nonspecialized nurses made malpractice payments in cases reported to NPDB, 1995–2001. Annual reports of the NPDB are available at www.npdb-hipdb.com. The author states that the majority of payments by nonspecialized nurses in malpractice suits resulted from problems relating to monitoring, treatment, medication, obstetrics, and surgery. Negligence areas discussed include failure to act as a patient advocate; failure to communicate adequate information to the physician or patient; inadequate patient assessment, nursing interventions, or nursing care; medication errors; inadequate infection control; failure to document; and unsafe or improper use of equipment. Monetary awards were paid either directly by independent practitioners or by employers according to the doctrine of respondeat superior. The author also discusses strategies for reducing potential liability.

**Implications for Practice:** Knowledge of the legal implications of nursing practice is necessary to assure that you are taking action to reduce your liability.

**Documentation.**    For protection when charting, the nurse should use the FLAT (Factual, Legible, Accurate, and Timely) charting acronym. See Table 5-6.

## Patient Advocacy and Ethical Behavior

Nursing's role as a patient advocate and follower of ethical behavior can help the nurse avoid being named in a lawsuit as well as help the nurse maintain quality nursing care. Nurses often intervene on behalf of the patient in the implementation of health care in areas such as notifying a nursing or medical practitioner of a patient problem, scheduling of treatment by other departments, appropriate referrals, explaining how the system works, assisting with follow-up activities, reinforcement of health teaching, coordination of care, preparation for safe discharge, and notification of appropriate individuals.

**TABLE 5-6**
*FLAT CHARTING*

F: Charting should be Factual—what you see, not what you think happened.

L: Charting should be Legible, with no erasures. Corrections should be made with a single line drawn through the error and initialed.

A: Charting should be Accurate and complete. What color was the drainage and how much was present? How many times, and at what times, was the doctor notified of changes?

T: Charting should be Timely, completed as soon after the occurrence as possible. Late entries should be avoided or kept to a minimum.

The nurse plays a unique role in the delivery of health care in acting as the intermediary between the patient and the health care system. The nurse is often the key person involved in identifying a patient problem and ensuring the patient access to appropriate quality health care. Nurses who advocate for their patient, maintain good communication with them and follow ethical principles and rules in an ethical workplace will have little problem with malpractice. See Table 5-7 & Table 5-8.

# Risk Management Programs

Risk management programs in health care organizations are designed to identify and correct system problems that contribute to errors in patient care or to employee injury. The emphasis in risk management programs is on quality improvement and protection of the institution from financial liability. Institutions usually have reporting and tracking forms that record incidents that may lead to financial liability for the institution. Risk management will assist in identifying and correcting the underlying problem that may have led to an incident, such as faulty equipment, staffing or delegation concerns, or the need for a better orientation for employees. Once a system problem is identified the Risk Management Department may develop strategies and educational programs for health care staff to address the problem.

The Risk Management Department may also investigate and record information surrounding a patient or employee incident that may result in a lawsuit. This helps personnel remember critical factors if called to testify at a later time. The nurse should notify the Risk Management Department of all reportable incidents and complete all Risk Management and/or Incident Report forms as mandated by institutional policies and procedures. Note that

## TABLE 5-7
## *ETHICAL PRINCIPLES AND RULES*

| Ethical Principle/Rule | Definition | Example |
|---|---|---|
| Beneficence | The duty to do good to others and to maintain a balance between benefits and harms. | • Provide all patients, including the terminally ill, with caring attention and information.<br>• Become familiar with your state laws regarding organ donations.<br>• Treat every patient with respect and courtesy. |
| Nonmaleficence | The principle of doing no harm. | • Always work within your scope of practice.<br>• Never give information or perform duties you are not qualified to do.<br>• Observe all safety rules and precautions.<br>• Keep areas safe from hazards.<br>• Perform procedures according to facility protocols. Never take shortcuts.<br>• Ask an appropriate person about anything you are unsure of.<br>• Keep your skills and education up to date. |
| Justice | The principle of fairness that is served when an individual is given that which he or she is due, owed, deserves, or can legitimately claim. | • Treat all patients equally, regardless of economic or social background.<br>• Learn the local, state, and national laws and your facility's policies and procedures for handling and reporting suspected abuse. |
| Autonomy and Confidentiality | Respect for an individual's right to self-determination; respect for individual liberty and privacy. | • Be sure that patients have consented to all treatments and procedures. |

*(continues)*

**Table 5-7** (*continued*)

| Ethical Principle/Rule | Definition | Example |
|---|---|---|
| | | • Become familiar with federal and state laws and facility policies dealing with privacy, e.g., HIPPA legislation. <br> • Never release patient information of any kind unless there is a signed patient release. <br> • Do not discuss patients with anyone who is not professionally involved in their care. <br> • Protect the physical privacy of patients. |
| **Fidelity** | The principle of promise keeping; the duty to keep one's promise or word. | • Be sure that contracts have been completed. <br> • Be very careful about what you say to patients. They may only hear the "good news." |
| **Respect for others** | The right of people to make their own decision. | • Provide all persons with information for decision making. <br> • Avoid making paternalistic decisions for others. |
| **Veracity** | The obligation to tell the truth. | • Admit mistakes promptly. Offer to do whatever is necessary to correct them. <br> • Refuse to participate in any form of fraud. <br> • Give an "honest day's work" every day. |
| **Advocacy** | The obligation to look out or speak up for the rights of others. | • Provide patients with high quality, evidence-based care. |

**TABLE 5-8**
*CREATING AN ETHICAL WORKPLACE*

Establishing an ethical and socially responsible workplace is not simply a matter of luck and common sense. Nurse managers can develop strategies and programs to enhance ethical and socially responsible attitudes. These may include:

1. Formal mechanisms for monitoring ethics, such as an ethics program or ethics hotline.
2. Written organizational codes of conduct.
3. Widespread communication in the hospital to reinforce ethically and socially responsible behavior.
4. Leadership by example: if people throughout the firm believe that behaving ethically is "in" and behaving unethically is "out," ethical behavior will prevail.
5. Encouraging confrontation about ethical deviations. Unethical behavior may be minimized if every employee confronts anyone seen behaving unethically.
6. Training programs in ethics and social responsibility, including messages about ethics from executives, classes on ethics at colleges, and exercises in ethics (DuBrin, 2000).
7. Instituting an ethics committee made up of interdisciplinary representatives from nursing, medicine, administration, clergy, consumers, psychiatry, social work, nutritional services, pharmacy, as well as an ethicist. Additional persons may be invited on an as needed basis. Ethical dilemmas may be referred to the ethics committee by anyone. This committee provides guidance to patients, families, and the health care team.

employee complaints of harassment or discrimination can expose the institution to significant liability and should promptly be reported to supervisors and the Risk Management Department, to Human Resources, or another department as specified in the institution's policies. The Risk Management Department staff also participate on key hospital committees, such as the Patient Safety Committee, Environment of Care Committee, Pharmacy and Nursing Committee, Ethics Committee, and other hospital committees which work on proactive programs to reduce risks (Martin & Cain, 2003). See Table 5-9 for a nursing checklist of actions to decrease the risk of nursing liability.

## Malpractice/Professional Liability Insurance

Nurses often wonder if they should carry their own malpractice insurance. Nurses may think their actions are adequately covered by the employer's lia-

## TABLE 5-9
### NURSING CHECKLIST OF ACTIONS TO DECREASE LIABILITY

- Use the National Council of State Boards of Nursing (NCSBN) Delegation Decision-Making Grid or your agency's delegation grid to make safe delegation decisions.
- Delegate patient care based on patients' needs, staff competency and skill, and the documented education, skill, and experience of licensed and unlicensed personnel.
- Develop a professional, assertive communication style with nursing and medical staff to assist you with meeting patient care goals.
- Identify realistic, attainable outcome standards to use to identify completion of any task that is delegated. Make frequent walking rounds to assure quality patient outcomes after delegation.
- Treat all patients and their families with kindness and respect.
- Take appropriate actions to meet the patient's nursing needs.
- Communicate with your patients and keep them informed.
- Communicate the patient's name, room number, and expectations for staff before, during, and after duty performance in a pleasant, direct, and concise manner when delegating patient care.
- Acknowledge unfortunate incidents and express concern about these events without either taking the blame, blaming others, or reacting defensively.
- Promptly report any concern regarding the quality of care, including the lack of resources with which to provide care, faulty equipment, staffing concerns, medication concerns, orientation or education concerns, complaints of discrimination or harassment, and patient or family complaints to a nursing administration representative.
- Follow evidence-based standards of care and the facility's policy and procedure for administering care and reporting incidents. Document the reason for any omission or deviation from the standards.
- Maintain current professional standards of care and clinical competency. Acknowledge your limitations. If you do not know how to do something, ask for help.
- Assume personal responsibility to develop professional educational certifications and clinical expertise.
- Avoid taking telephone and verbal orders. If needed, repeat the order back to the practitioner to assure clarity. Document that you did this, e.g., telephone order repeated back (TORB) or verbal order repeated back (VORB).
- Encourage the development of clearly written and/or computerized orders from all practitioners.
- Chart and time your observations immediately, while facts are still fresh in your mind.

*(continues)*

**Table 5-9** (*continued*)

- Document the time of nursing actions and changes in conditions requiring notification of the physician. Include the response of the physician. Use the chain of command at your agency to report any concerns.
- Complete incident reports immediately after they occur. Discuss critical factors with the risk manager to increase your retention of the facts.
- Follow professional guidelines for safe transfer of all patients both inside and outside the agency.

bility insurance but this is not necessarily so. While the hospital's insurance company almost always pays malpractice awards, insurance contracts often have provisions that allow them to refuse payment if the insured intentionally injures another party (Pozza, 2003). Also, if in giving care, the nurse fails to comply with the institution's policies and procedures, the institution may deny the nurse a defense, claiming that because of the nurse's failure to follow institutional policy the nurse was not acting as an employee at that time. Nurses are also being named individually as defendants in malpractice suits more frequently than was the case in the past although hospitals are often a plaintiff's primary target because they typically have deeper pockets than individual practitioners (Pozza, 2003). It is advantageous for the nurse to be assured of a defense independent of that of his or her employer. Professional liability insurance provides that assurance and pays for an attorney to defend the nurse in a malpractice lawsuit.

Note that in the event that an unaffiliated nurse, like an agency per diem nurse, is held individually liable for a judgment, the nurse's personal insurance carrier will be responsible for paying the verdict rendered against the nurse. An unaffiliated, uninsured nurse could be forced to pay for her own defense and be financially responsible for any judgments rendered against her.

In making the decision of whether to obtain separate insurance, a nurse should consider the value of their personal assets. A nurse should also consider the laws of the state in which they practice regarding those assets that are exempt from being seized to satisfy civil monetary judgments. Generally, one home and one automobile are exempt from seizure (Pozza, 2003).

# NURSING RISK IN LITIGATION

Nurses may be sued individually for damages resulting from their negligent acts.[13] [15] [16] [18] [23] [30] [38] [44] However, often a plaintiff will name the nurse's employer as a defendant instead of, or in addition to, suing the nurse individually. In other words, a hospital, nursing home, or clinic, is often held legally responsible for the damages caused by the negligence of its nurses. It is well-established law throughout the United States that "a master is subject to liability for the torts of his servants committed while acting in the scope of employment."[51] This law is called Respondeat Superior. It is set out in the Restatement of the Law of Agency. The Restatement sets forth principles of common law that are generally accepted in all courts throughout the country. Respondeat Superior is one such law.

A plaintiff may also sue the hospital, nursing home, or health clinic for its direct negligence. For example, nursing homes have been sued for failing to adequately train and supervise personnel.[8 19 24 34] Hospitals have been sued for allowing unlicensed personnel to administer medications[34] and for failing to provide appropriate laboratory services to patients.[23] Hospitals may also be held legally responsible for failing to maintain appropriate policies and procedures regarding staffing, quality assurance, and chain of command (Pozza, 2003).

In many malpractice cases involving hospitals, the physicians involved are also named individually.[1 3 6 7 11 12 13 21 24 26 28 33 34 37 40 41 43] Customarily, plaintiffs in medical malpractice cases name a combination of health care providers as defendants. It is common for some or all of the defendants to settle the cases before they reach the trial phase. However, in the event that a case proceeds to trial, a jury may find that none, some, or all of the defendants were negligent in their care and treatment of the plaintiff. A jury may determine that the nursing care was appropriate, but the medical treatment was substandard. Likewise, a jury could hold that the physician rendered appropriate care, but the nurses' conduct fell below the standard of care. Additionally, a new trend in malpractice litigation is to name the Health Maintenance Organization (HMO) as a defendant as well. For example, the Illinois Supreme Court recently held that a HMO could be liable under theories of apparent authority, respondeat superior, direct corporate negligence, breach of contract, and breach of warranty[49] (Pozza, 2003).

President Bush recently announced his plan to encourage federal legislation limiting punitive damages in medical malpractice lawsuits. Bush endorsed a bill in which the amount of punitive damages available in medical malpractice cases throughout the country could not exceed two times the amount of economic damages or $250,000, whichever is greater (Pozza, 2003).

## Common Monetary Awards

Many health care malpractice cases are dismissed or settled prior to trial. In those cases that do reach the trial stage, jury verdicts are unpredictable and awards can vary dramatically. For instance, juries awarded the following for the listed injuries:

- brachial plexus injury ($13.3 million)[6]
- wrongful death—pulmonary embolism ($5 million)[1]
- microcephaly in newborn ($17 million)[11]
- vision loss ($8 million)[13]
- arterial impairment ($260,000)[52]

A jury may award the plaintiff both compensatory and punitive damages. Compensatory damages are awarded to compensate the plaintiff for his injuries. Compensatory damages include damages for both economic losses (medical expenses, lost wages, lost earning capacity) and non-economic losses (pain and suffering).

Punitive damages are not intended to compensate the plaintiff for any loss. Rather, punitive damages are intended to punish the defendant for acting with "recklessness, malice or deceit."[57] Punitive damage awards are particularly common in cases involving nursing homes. For example, a Texas jury awarded the family of a nursing home resident $90 million in punitive damages for gross negligence that caused the resident to develop pressure ulcers and contractures[50] (Pozza, 2003).

**Selected Monetary Liability Limits.**   Since 1970, at least 30 states have enacted legislation capping the monetary damages plaintiffs can recover in a lawsuit.[54] Currently, there exist as many different cap schemes as states that employ them. Some states cap the amount that a plaintiff may receive for punitive damages. See Table 5-10.

Other states employ a flat dollar cap. These states limit the total monetary amount the plaintiff may recover in both compensatory and punitive damages in any malpractice action. See Table 5-11.

A plaintiff may claim he or she is entitled to damages in excess of the applicable cap. Jurors are customarily not informed of the caps applicable in their states. Therefore, it is common for a jury's award to exceed the state's cap on damages. In the event that a jury awards a plaintiff damages in excess of a statutory cap, the judge will reduce the jury's award to the cap (Pozza, 2003).

# Other Legal Risks for the Nurse/Practitioner/Hospital

Other than increased insurance premiums, health care providers have much at stake when named as defendants in malpractice cases. Physicians are required to report adverse verdicts and settlements to the National Practitioner's Data Bank. The National Practitioner's Data Bank was established through the Health Care Quality Improvement Act of 1986. The federal regulations regarding the Data Bank can be found in 45 Code of Federal Regulations (CFR) Part 60. Significant awards against a physician or numerous malpractice payments by a physician can affect the physician's licensure or ability to gain privileges to practice at certain hospitals and health care enti-

## TABLE 5-10
### PUNITIVE DAMAGE LIMITS

| State | Punitive Damages limited to: |
| --- | --- |
| Alabama | $250,000 |
| Alaska | Three times compensatory damages or $500,000, whichever is greater |
| California | $500,000 |
| Georgia | $250,000 |
| Illinois | $5 million or the highest annual gross income earned by the defendant within the past five years, whichever is less |
| Kansas | $5 million or the highest annual gross income earned by the defendant within the past five years, whichever is less |
| Nevada | $300,000 (when compensatory damages are less than $100,000) |
| North Dakota | Twice the compensatory damages or $250,000, whichever is greater |
| Virginia | $350,000 |

Pozza, 2003

## TABLE 5-11
### SELECTED STATES WITH FLAT DOLLAR CAP ON LIABILITY

| State | Total verdict limited to: |
| --- | --- |
| Colorado | $1 million per patient |
| Nebraska | $1.25 million per patient |

Pozza, 2004

ties. Failure to report malpractice payments to the Data Bank can result in civil monetary penalties. The U.S. Department of Health and Human Services, Office of the Inspector General, may impose a civil money penalty of up to $11,000 for each violation.

Federal and state statutes and regulations prescribe nursing standards of care. See the Code of Federal Regulations Title 42-Public Health and Title 45-Public Welfare. See also U.S. Code Title 42-Public Health and Welfare.

Every jurisdiction that licenses nurses has a nurse practice act.[53] In addition to instructing nurses on the definition of the standard of care for that jurisdiction, the nurse practice act mandates strict rules for reporting and disciplining nurses who violate the standard. Likewise, state boards of nursing and administrative agencies may take action to suspend or revoke the licenses of nurses that it determines have violated the standard of care. Private entities, such as the Joint Commission on Accreditation of Healthcare Organizations (JCAHO), and professional organizations, such as the American Nurses Association (ANA), promulgate their own rules of conduct that serve as guidelines for acceptable nursing care (Pozza, 2003).

# NURSE-ATTORNEY RELATIONSHIP IN A LAWSUIT

In spite of the nurse's best intentions, a nurse may be named as a defendant in a lawsuit and need to retain the services of an attorney. LaDuke (2000) makes the following suggestions for consulting and collaborating with an attorney:

1. Retain a legal specialist. Generalist lawyers are competent to handle many matters, but professional malpractice, professional disciplinary proceedings, and employment disputes are best handled by specialists in those areas.
2. Be attentive. Read the documents the attorney produces and travel to court proceedings to observe the attorney's performance.
3. Notify your insurance carrier as soon as you are aware of any real or potential liability issue. Inform your agent about the status of your case every few months, even if it's unchanged.
4. Keep costs sensible. Your attorney should explain initially how the fee will be computed and how you will be billed. The attorney may require you to pay a retainer fee.
5. Keep informed. The attorney should address your questions and concerns promptly. You are entitled to be kept informed about the status of your case. You are entitled to copies of all correspondence, legal briefs, and other documents.
6. Weed through writing. Your attorney needs to explain all facts and options. Examine all relevant documents and do not hesitate to make corrections in the same way you would correct a medical record by drawing a line through the incorrect or misleading information, writing in the correction, and signing your initials after it.
7. Set your own course. Insist on a collaborative relationship with your attorney for the duration of your case.

# REVIEW QUESTIONS

1. An intentional false communication, either published or spoken, is which of the following?
   A. Assault
   B. Defamation
   C. Malpractice
   D. False Imprisonment

2. Invasion of privacy is an example of which of the following? Commission of:
   A. A tort
   B. An administrative law violation
   C. A Good Samaritan Law violation
   D. A criminal law violation

3. When there is a connection between the nurse breaching a duty and the damages occurring to a patient, this is an example of which of the following?
   A. Breach of duty
   B. Duty
   C. Causation
   D. Damages

4. Select the most appropriate documentation example below.
   A. Patient found covered in stool. The night nurses were too busy to change the bed.
   B. The patient fell because we are short of staff.
   C. The patient's family is difficult and argumentative.
   D. Doctor M. Bresley notified through the medical exchange at 0610 of patient's complaints of difficulty breathing. Orders received for oxygen and ABG's.

5. You call the attending physician for your new postoperative patient who is bleeding excessively. The patient's blood pressure has decreased by 20 mm Hg and the pulse rate has increased by 20 beats over the past hour. The physician's response to this information is, "Why did you wake me up at 2 A.M. for this? I am hanging up as I expect a postoperative patient to be oozing from the operative site and these changes are not significant. Just watch him." You are quite concerned about your patient. What will you do next?
   A. Go to the nursing station and complain to the other nurses about how rude the physician was on the phone.
   B. Document and quote the physician's response in your nurses notes.
   C. Inform the physician that you do not agree with continuing to just observe this patient and that you are going to initiate the chain of command.
   D. Tell the family what the physician said.

6. An 80-year-old male who lives with his son is brought to your unit because "he isn't acting right." On physical examination, you note that the patient is malnourished, non-communicative, and has poor hygiene. When asking the patient some questions, he avoids eye contact and does not respond. The son is answering questions for the patient and refuses to leave the room. You suspect elder abuse. Choose the most appropriate documentation of the situation.

   A. The patient is very thin and does not make eye contact with the nursing or medical staff. It is obvious that he has been abused and neglected by his family.

   B. The patient is a thin elderly male who presents to the unit wearing clothing that is soiled. He does not make eye contact with the staff or answer our questions. Social services notified.

   C. It appears that the patient's son manipulates his father by refusing to let his father answer any questions. We suspect elder abuse.

   D. The patient's son states that the patient "isn't acting right." The patient does not answer questions from the staff due to his abuse.

## REVIEW ACTIVITIES

1. Talk to the Risk Manager at a hospital where you have your clinical assignments. Ask him to comment on which hospital committees he serves. How does the Risk Management Department and other hospital committees work to decrease hospital liability and improve patient care?

2. You are working the night shift. One of the physicians has ordered a dose of a medication to be given to your patient that you know is too high for this patient. You are unable to locate the physician to check the order. What would you do to assure safe care for your patient?

## EXPLORING THE WEB

1. Check this site for state and federal laws regulating hospitals.
   www.findlaw.com

2. Find a copy of the ANA code of Ethics at
   www.ana.org
   Search for "code of ethics"

3. Check these sites for ANA position papers
   http://www.nursingworld.org
   and click on position statements. Note various positions on the role of the nurse. Also note information about magnet hospitals and risk management that can be accessed through this site.

4. Note the information available at
   http://www.ncsbn.org

5. The Code of Federal Regulations is available at the United States Government Printing Office website
   http://www.access.gpo.gov

6. The United States Code is available at the Office of the Law Revision Counsel website
   http://uscode.house.gov/uscode.htm

7. Find legal research at the Law and Policy Institutions Guide
   www.lpig.org

8. Check the information you can find at these sites:
   www.westlaw.com
   www.lexis.com
   www.aslme.com
   www.jcaho.org
   www.cms.hhs.gov

## REFERENCES

Croke, E. M. (2003). Nurses, negligence, and malpractice. *American Journal of Nursing, 103*(9), 54–64.

Fiesta, J. (1999, August). Do no harm: When caregivers violate our golden rule, Part 1. *Nursing Management, Volume 30,* 10–11.

Garner, B., Black, H. C., & Garner, B. A. (2001). *Black's Law Dictionary.* Ann Arbor, MI: West Group Publishing.

LaDuke, S. (2000, January). What should you expect from your attorney? *Nursing Management, Volume 31,* 10.

Martin, J., & Cain, K. (2003). In P. Kelly-Heidenthal. Nursing leadership and management. Clifton Park, NY: Delmar.

Mitchell, P. R., & Grippando, G. M. (1993). Nursing perspectives and issues. Clifton Park, NY: Delmar.

Pozza, R. (2003). Legal aspects of nursing. Unpublished Manuscript. Austin, TX.

Zerwekh, J., & Claborn, J. (2002). Nursing today. Transition and trends. St. Louis, MO: Saunders.

## SUGGESTED READINGS

Carson, W. Y. (2001). Nursing malpractice: protect yourself. *American Journal of Nursing, 101*(12), 81.

Fiesta, J. (1999, July). Informed consent: What health care professionals need to know, Part 2. *Nursing Management, Volume 30,* 6–7.

Fiesta, J. (1999, September). Know your boundaries in sexual assault litigation. *Nursing Management, Volume 30,* 10.

Fiesta, J. (1999, November). Greater need for background checks. *Nursing Management, Volume 30,* 26.

Giordano, K. (2003). Examining nursing malpractice: a defense attorney's perspective. *Critical Care Nurse, 23*(2), 104–108.

Guido, G. W. (2001). Legal and ethical issues in nursing. Upper Saddle River, NJ: Prentice Hall.

Landry, H., & Landry, M. (2002). Nursing ethics and legal issues: an integrative approach in nursing education. *Journal of Nursing Education, 41*(8), 363–364.

Mayberry, A., & Croke, E. (1996). Issues leading to malpractice show little change: A review of the literature. Journal of Legal Nurse Consulting, *7*(2), 16–19.

Michael, J. E. (2002). Expert witnessing brings nursing expertise into the legal arena. *Nursing Management, 33*(3), 23–24, 56.

O'Keefe, M. E. (2001). *Nursing practice and the law.* Philadelphia: F. A. Davis Company.

Sloan, A. J. (1999, July). Legally speaking: Whistleblowing: there are risks! *Registered Nurse, Volume 62,* 65–66, 68.

Sheehan, J. P. (2000, March). Protect your staff from workplace violence. *Nursing Management, Volume 31,* 24–25.

Smith-Pitman, M. (1998). Nurses and litigation: 1990–1997. *Journal of Nursing Law, 5*(2), 7–19.

Sullivan, G. H. (1999, April). Legally speaking: Minimizing your risk in patient falls. *Registered Nurse, 62,* 69–70, 72.

Sullivan, G. H. (2000, May). Legally speaking: Keep your charting on course. *Registered Nurse, 63,* 75–79.

## CASE REFERENCES

1. *Martinelli v. Lifemark Hosps. of Fla., Inc.,* Fla., Dade County Cir. Ct., No. 99-14491 CA 05, Mar. 1, 2001. 16 *ATLA* PNLR 111, July 2001.

2. *Doe v. Roe Hosp.,* Ohio, Cuyahoga County C.C.P., confidential docket number, Feb. 2001. 16 *PNLR* 113, July 2001.

3. *Montalvo v. Mercy Hosp.*, Tex., Webb County 111th Jud. Dist. Ct., No. 98-CVQ-01126-D2, Aug. 4, 2000. 16 *PNLR* 116, July 2001.

4. *Doe v. Roe,* confidential state, court, and docket number, Dec. 2000. 16 *PNLR* 117, July 2001.

5. *Fuqua v. Horizon/CMS Healthcare Corp.*, U.S. Dist. Ct., N.D. Tex., No. 4-98-CV-1087-Y, Feb. 14, 2001. 16 *PNLR* 117, July 2001.

6. *Stonieczny v. Gardner,* Ill., Cook County Cir. Ct., No. 98 L 04578, May 29, 2001. 16 *PNLR* 131, Sept 2001.

7. *Doe v. Roe,* N.C., confidential court and docket number, Dec. 4, 2000. 16 *PNLR* 137, Sept 2001.

8. *Nash v. Compton Mgmt., Inc.,* Ark., Cross County Cir. Ct., No. CIV-99-34, June 7, 2001. 16 *PNLR* 137, Sept 2001.

9. *Copeland v. Dallas Home for Jewish Aged, Inc.,* Tex., Dallas County 134th Jud. Dist. Ct., No. 98-04690, May 21, 2001. 16 *PNLR* 138, Sept 2001.

10. *Doe v. Kimberly QualityCare, Inc.,* Ariz., Maricopa County Super. Ct., No. CV-96-10499, June 1, 2001. 16 *PNLR* 149, Oct 2001.

11. *Diver v. Gingo,* Ohio, Cuyahoga County C.C.P., No. 305538, Jan. 2001. 16 *PNLR* 152, Oct 2001.

12. *Williams v. Hospital Auth. of Valdosta,* U.S. Dist. Ct., M.D. Ga., No. 7:98-CV-79(WDO), Dec. 23, 2000. 16 *PNLR* 152, Oct 2001.

13. *Schwab v. Kamat,* N.Y., Onondaga County Sup. Ct., No. 97-887, June 8, 2001. 16 *PNLR* 154, Oct 2001.

14. *Furman v. San Pedro Peninsula Hosp.,* Cal., Los Angeles County Super. Ct., No. NC025678, Feb. 28, 2001. 16 *PNLR* 154, Oct 2001.

15. *Marshal v. Methodist Healthcare Jackson Hosp.,* Miss., Hinds County Cir. Ct., No. 251-99-000984CIV, Jan. 23, 2001. 16 *PNLR* 174, Nov 2001.

16. *Lewis v. Physicians Ins. Co. of Wis.,* 627 N.W.2d 484 (Wis. 2001). 16 *PNLR* 175, Nov 2001.

17. *Doe v. Roe Med. Group,* Ohio, Richland County C.C.P., confidential docket no., Mar. 20, 2001. 16 *PNLR* 176, Nov 2001.

18. *Doe v. Roe,* confidential court and docket no., Apr. 2001. 16 *PNLR* 177, Nov 2001.

19. *Sauer v. Advocat, Inc.,* Ark., Polk County Cir. Ct., No. CIV-2000-5, June 22, 2001. 16 *PNLR* 179, Nov 2001.

20. *Johnson v. Commonwealth of Virginia,* Va., Stafford County Cir. Ct., No. 99191, Apr. 2001. 16 *PNLR* 197, Dec 2001.

21. *Couch v. St. Luke's Med. Ctr. RMC,* Idaho, Ada County Dist. Ct., Nos. 9900289D, 99000358D, May 2001. 16 *PNLR* 197, Dec 2001.

22. *Doe v. United States,* confidential court and docket no., 2001. 16 *PNLR* 200, Dec 2001.

23. *Urgent v. Government of the Virgin Islands,* U.S.V.I., V.I. Territorial Ct. St. Croix Div., No. 607/1998, Sept. 13, 2001. 17 *PNLR* 8, Feb 2002.

24. *Johns v. Franciscan Health Sys.W.,* Wash., King County Super. Ct., No. 99-2-04211-5KNT, Oct. 30, 2001. 17 *PNLR* 9, Feb 2002.
25. *Doe v. Sibley Hosp.,* D.C., D.C. Super. Ct., No. 983387, Aug. 16, 2001. 17 *PNLR* 9, Feb 2002.
26. *Chichy v. Ghate,* Pa., Indiana County C.C.P., No. 11048 CD 1997, June 25, 2001. 17 *PNLR* 10, Feb 2002.
27. *Arledge v. Oak Grove Nursing Home, Inc.,* Tex., Jefferson County 58th Jud. Dist. Ct., No. A162668, Sept. 18, 2001. 17 *PNLR* 11, Feb 2002.
28. *Lee v. Chen,* Ill., Cook County Cir. Ct., No. 95 L 2796, Sept. 27, 2001. 17 *PNLR* 28, Mar 2002.
29. *Graham v. Forrest Gen. Hosp.,* Miss., Forrest County Cir. Ct., No. CI00-0165, June 12, 2001. 17 *PNLR* 31, Mar 2002.
30. *Lavalis v. Copperas Cove L.L.C.,* Tex., Bell County 146th Jud. Dist. Ct., No. 183,293-B, Dec. 27, 2001. 17 *PNLR* 32, Mar 2002.
31. *Doe v. Roe Nursing Home,* U.S. Dist. Ct., D. Kan., No. 99-1474WEB, Aug. 2001. 17 *PNLR* 32, Mar 2002.
32. *Stevens v. Contra Costa Reg'l Med. Ctr.,* Cal., settled before filing, Dec. 17, 2001. 17 *PNLR* 46, Apr 2002.
33. *Doe v. Roe,* Md., confidential court, docket no., and date. 17 *PNLR* 48, Apr 2002.
34. *Solomon v. Desert Valley Hosp., Inc.,* Cal., San Bernardino County Super. Ct., No. VCV017352, Sept. 10, 2001. 17 *PNLR* 51, Apr 2002.
35. *Palmer v. South Ala. Nursing Homes, Inc.,* Ala., Mobile County Cir. Ct., No. CV002775, Dec. 14, 2001. 17 *PNLR* 52, Apr 2002.
36. *Johnson v. Weiss Mem'l Hosp.,* Ill., Cook County Cir. Ct., No. 01 L 6581, Mar. 13, 2002. 17 *PNLR* 66, May 2002.
37. *Doe v. Roe,* N.C., confidential court and docket no., Dec. 18, 2001. 17 *PNLR* 66, May 2002.
38. *Huckaby v. Lake Pointe Partners, LTD.,* Tex., Rockwall County 382d Jud. Dist. Ct., No. 1-00-592, Dec. 14, 2001. 17 *PNLR* 67, May 2002.
39. *Doe v. Roe,* N.C., confidential court and docket no., Jan. 2002. 17 *PNLR* 68, May 2002.
40. *Nunn v. Galen of Ky., Inc.,* Ky., Jefferson County Cir. Ct., No. 97-CI-05753, Oct. 1, 2001. 17 *PNLR* 69, May 2002.
41. *Moore v. Allegheny Univ. Hosp.-City Ave.,* Pa., Phila. County C.C.P., No. 980602267, Jan. 14, 2002. 17 *PNLR* 70, May 2002.
42. *Doe v. Roe,* Md., Baltimore City Cir. Ct., confidential docket no., June 14, 2001. 17 *PNLR* 71, May 2002.
43. *Doe v. Roe,* Cal., Los Angeles County Super. Ct., confidential docket no., Dec. 2001. 17 *PNLR* 71, May 2002.
44. *Boze v. Universal Nursing Servs. Ltd.,* Fla., Hernando County Cir. Ct., No. H-27-CA-2001-1706, Mar. 21, 2002. 17 *PNLR* 104, July 2002.

45. *M.N. v. Variety Children's Hosp.,* Fla., Dade County Cir. Ct., No. 98-16750 CA 06, Dec. 19, 2001. 17 *PNLR* 108, July 2002.
46. *Washington v. Kings Daughters Hosp.,* Miss., Washington County Cir. Ct., No. C197-0130, Mar. 28, 2002. 17 *PNLR* 110, July 2002.
47. *Mays v. Palestine Principal Healthcare L.P.,* Tex., Anderson County 349th Jud. Dist. Ct., No. 4744, Feb. 22, 2002. 17 *PNLR* 111, July 2002.
48. Hyman, David A. (2002) Medical Malpractice and the Tort System: What Do We Know and What (If Anything) Should We Do About It? 80 Tex.L.Rev. 1639.
49. *Jones v. ChicagoHMO Ltd. Of Ill.,* 730 N.E.2d 1119 (Ill. 2000).
50. *Horizon/CMS Healthcare Corp. v. Auld,* 34 S.W.3d 887 (Tex. 2000).
51. Restatement (Second) of the Law of Agency §219 (1958).
52. *In re Triss,* 2002 WL 1271492 (La.App. 4 Cir., 2002).
53. Cavico, Frank J. and Cavico, Nancy M. (1995) The Nursing Profession in the 1990s: Negligence and Malpractice Liability. 43 Clev. St. L. Rev. 557.
54. Babcock, Linda and Pogarsky, Greg. (1999) Damages Caps and Settlement: A Behavioral Approach. 28 Journal of Legal Studies 341.
55. *Darling v. Charleston Comm. Mem. Hosp.,* 211 N.E.2d 253 (Ill. 1965).
56. *Suburban Hospital, Inc. v. Kirson,* 763 A.2d 185 (Md. 2000).
57. Black's Law Dictionary 396 (7th ed. 1999).

# GLOSSARY

**Accountability**   Being responsible and answerable for actions or inactions of self or others in the context of delegation.

**Activity log**   Time management tool that can assist the nurse in determining how both personal and professional time is used.

**Anger**   A universal, strong feeling of displeasure that is often precipitated by a situation that frustrates or prevents a person from attaining a goal.

**Assignment**   The downward or lateral transfer of both the responsibility and accountability of an activity from one individual to another.

**Attending**   Activity involving active listening.

**Authority**   The right to act or to command the action of others.

**Blaming**   Finding fault or error, this occurs when a response lacks respect for others' feelings.

**Civil law**   Law that affects the relationship between individuals.

**Clarifying**   Communication that becomes clear through the use of such techniques as restating and questioning.

**Communication**   The sending and receiving of a message.

**Confronting**   Working jointly with others or to resolve a problem or conflict.

**Critical thinking**   Indicates "thinking about your thinking while you're thinking in order to make your thinking better."

**Delegation**   The transfer of responsibility for the performance of an activity from one individual to another while retaining accountability for the outcome.

**Good Samaritan Laws**   Laws that have been enacted to protect the health care professional from legal liability for actions rendered in an emergency when the professional is giving service without pay.

**Indirect patient care**   Activities often necessary to support the patient and their environment, and only incidentally involve direct patient contact.

**Malpractice** A professional's wrongful conduct in discharge of their professional duties or failure to meet standards of care for the profession which results in harm to another individual entrusted to the nurse's care.

**Negligence** The failure to provide the care a reasonable person would ordinarily provide in a similar situation.

**Nursing judgment** The process by which nurses come to understand the problems, issues, or concerns of clients, to attend to salient information, and to respond to client problems in concerned and involved ways.

**Pareto principle** When 20% of focused effort results in 80% of desired outcomes or results, or conversely when 80% of unfocused effort results in 20% of results.

**Responding** Verbal and nonverbal acknowledgment of the sender's message.

**Responsibility** Obligations involved when one accepts an assignment.

**Supervision** Providing of guidance or direction, evaluation, and follow-up by the licensed nurse for the accomplishment of a nursing task delegated to UAP.

**Time management** A set of related common-sense skills that helps you use your time in the most effective and productive way possible.

**Tort** A private or civil wrong or injury, including action for bad faith breach of contract, for which the court will provide a remedy in the form of an action for damages.

# INDEX